Procedure Check
Fundamentals of Nursing

Judith M. Wilkinson, PhD, ARNP

Nurse-Educator/Consultant

Shawnee, Kansas

Karen Van Leuven, PhD, FNP

Associate Professor

University of San Francisco

San Francisco, California

Family Nurse Practitioner

Oakland, California

F.A. Davis Company • Philadelphia

F. A. Davis Company
1915 Arch Street
Philadelphia, PA 19103
www.fadavis.com

Printed in the United States of America

Last digit indicates print number: 10 9 8 7 6 5 4 3

ISBN 13: 978-0-8036-1473-4
ISBN 10: 0-8036-1473-X

Acquisitions Editor: Lisa B. Deitch
Developmental Editor: Shirley A. Kuhn
Senior Project Editor: Danielle J. Barsky
Content Development Manager: Darlene D. Pedersen

As new scientific information becomes available through basic and clinical research, recommended treatments and drug therapies undergo changes. The author(s) and publisher have done everything possible to make this book accurate, up to date, and in accord with accepted standards at the time of publication. The author(s), editors, and publisher are not responsible for errors or omissions or for consequences from application of the book, and make no warranty, expressed or implied, in regard to the contents of the book. Any practice described in this book should be applied by the reader in accordance with professional standards of care used in regard to the unique circumstances that may apply in each situation. The reader is advised always to check product information (package inserts) for changes and new information regarding dose and contraindications before administering any drug. Caution is especially urged when using new or infrequently ordered drugs.

Introduction

These checklists are designed for teachers to use when evaluating student skills and for students to use when practicing skills or participating in peer check-offs. There are two types of checklist:
* For each procedure, a checklist containing all the procedural steps, created specifically for that procedure.
* One principles-based checklist that applies to <u>all</u> procedures (see the inside back covers of this book and of Wilkinson and Van Leuven/*Fundamentals of Nursing: Thinking and Doing*, Vol. 2, F. A. Davis, 2007).

The principles checklist can be used in two ways:
1. For evaluating students, especially in clinical settings, teachers can use it <u>instead of</u> the steps-based checklists. If you choose, you can evaluate all procedures using this one piece of paper. Simply make as many copies as you need. For example, if you have 8 students and you expect to evaluate 3 skills per day, then you will need 24 copies for a clinical day.
2. For all students, and for teachers who prefer the individual, steps-based forms, you should use the principles checklist as the first page for each of those. Make as many copies of the principles checklist as you need.

Contents

PROCEDURE Checklist
Chapter 9: Assessing for Abuse

Check (✓)Yes or No

PROCEDURE STEPS	Yes	No	COMMENTS
1. If sexual abuse is suspected, has a forensic nurse or sexual assault nurse examiner (SANE) present, if possible.			
2. Uses a nonjudgmental approach. Does not make assumptions.			
3. Takes a health history.			
a. Assesses for physical abuse.			
b. Assesses for psychological abuse.			
c. Assesses for sexual abuse.			
d. Includes history of past injuries.			
e. Collects information from the patient and parents or caregivers separately.			
f. Phrases questions appropriately for age (child, adolescent, adult).			
4. Performs a physical assessment.			
a. Looks for bruises, circular burns, vaginal bleeding, poor sphincter tone, etc.			
b. Ensures the integrity of evidence that may be needed for criminal prosecution.			
5. Assesses whether injuries are consistent with history.			
6. Observes for signs of neglect (e.g., distended abdomen, poor hygiene, pressure sores, matted hair, underweight).			
7. If appropriate, refers for help in escaping the abusive situation.			
8. If appropriate, refers parent, caregiver, or partner involved in abuse to hotlines or agencies focused on stopping the abuse.			
9. Reports abuse according to agency and state guidelines.			

Recommendation: Pass _____ Needs more practice _____

Student: _____ Date: _____

Instructor: _____ Date: _____

PROCEDURE CHECKLIST
Chapter 10: Admitting a Patient to a Nursing Unit

Check (✓) Yes or No

PROCEDURE STEPS	Yes	No	COMMENTS
1. Introduces self to patient and family.			
2. Assists patient into hospital gown.			
3. If possible, measures weight while standing on a scale.			
4. Transfers patient to the bed.			
5. Checks patient's identification band to ensure information, including allergies, is correct. Verifies this information with the patient or family.			
6. Measures patient's vital signs.			
7. Explains equipment, including how to use call system and location of personal care items.			
8. Explains hospital routines, including use of side rails, meal times, etc., and answers patient's and family's questions.			
9. Obtains nursing admission assessment (including health history) and physical assessment.			
10. Completes inventory of patient's belongings. Encourages family to take home valuable items. If that is not possible, arranges to have valuables placed in the hospital safe.			
11. Ensures that all admission orders have been completed.			
12. Initiates care plan or clinical pathway.			
13. Documents all findings.			

Recommendation: Pass _____ Needs more practice _____

Student: _____ Date: _____

Instructor: _____ Date: _____

PROCEDURE CHECKLIST
Chapter 17: Assessing Body Temperature

Check (✓)Yes or No

PROCEDURE STEPS	Yes	No	COMMENTS
1. Selects appropriate site and thermometer type.			
2. "Zeroes" or shakes down glass thermometer as needed.			
3. Inserts thermometer in sheath or uses thermometer designated only for the patient.			
4. Inserts in chosen route/site. a. *Oral*: Places thermometer tip under the tongue in the posterior sublingual pocket (right or left of frenulum). Asks patient to keep lips closed. b. *Rectal*: Lubricates thermometer; uses rectal thermometer; inserts 1 to 1.5 inches (2.5–3.7 cm) in an adult; 0.9 inches (2.5 cm) for a child, and 0.5 inch (1.5 cm) for infant. c. *Axillary*: Dries axilla; Places thermometer tip in the middle of the axilla; lowers patient's arm. d. *Tympanic membrane*: Positions the patient's head to one side and straighten the ear canal. 1) For an adult, pulls the pinna up and back. 2) For a child, pull the pinna down and back			
5. Leaves glass thermometer recommended time (oral 3–5 min, rectal 2 min, axillary 6–8 min).			
6. Holds rectal thermometer securely in places; does not leave patient unattended.			
7. Leaves electronic thermometer until it beeps.			
8. Reads temperature. Holds glass thermometer at eye level to read.			
9. Shakes down (as needed) and cleans or stores thermometer.			

Recommendation: Pass _____ Needs more practice _____

Student: _____   Date: _____

Instructor: _____   Date: _____

PROCEDURE CHECKLIST
Chapter 17: Assessing Peripheral Pulses

Check (✓) Yes or No

PROCEDURE STEPS	Yes	No	COMMENTS
NOTE: You can use this checklist to evaluate one peripheral pulse, or to evaluate the student's ability to locate all the peripheral pulses.			

Circle site used:
    radial, brachial, carotid, temporal, popliteal, femoral,
    posterior tibial, dorsalis pedis			

1. Selects, correctly locates, and palpates site.			
2. Uses fingers (not thumb) to palpate.			
3. Counts for 30 sec. if regular; 60 sec. if irregular.			
4. Notes rate, rhythm, and quality.			
5. Compares bilaterally.			
6. Carotid pulse: Palpates only on one side at a time.			
7. Correctly locates the following sites: a. radial			
b. brachial			
c. carotid			
d. temporal			
e. popliteal			
f. femoral			
g. posterior tibial			
h. dorsalis pedis			

Recommendation: Pass _____ Needs more practice _____

Student: _____   Date: _____

Instructor: _____   Date: _____

Check (✓) Yes or No

PROCEDURE STEPS	Yes	No	COMMENTS
1. Flexes patient's arm and places patient's forearm across chest, or otherwise counts unobtrusively.			
2. Counts for 30 seconds if respirations regular; 60 seconds if irregular.			
3. Observes rate, rhythm, and depth.			

Recommendation: Pass _____ Needs more practice _____

Student: _____   Date: _____

Instructor: _____   Date: _____

PROCEDURE CHECKLIST
Chapter 17: Assessing the Apical Pulse

Check (✓) Yes or No

PROCEDURE STEPS	Yes	No	COMMENTS
1. Selects, correctly locates, and palpates apical site (5th intercostal space at the midclavicular line).			
2. Uses diaphragm of stethoscope.			
3. Counts for 60 seconds.			
4. Notes rate, rhythm, and quality.			
5. Identifies S1 and S2 heart sounds.			

Recommendation: Pass _____ Needs more practice _____

Student: _____   Date: _____

Instructor: _____   Date: _____

PROCEDURE CHECKLIST
Chapter 17: Assessing for an Apical-Radial Pulse Deficit

Check [✓] Yes or No

PROCEDURE STEPS	Yes	No	COMMENTS
1. Selects, correctly locates, and palpates apical site (5th intercostal space at the midclavicular line).			
2. Obtains another nurse to assist.			
3. Places watch so it is visible to both nurses.			
4. One nurse palpates radial pulse; the other uses diaphragm of stethoscope to auscultate the apex. Correctly locates sites.			
5. Counts for 60 seconds.			
6. Notes rate, rhythm, and quality.			
7. Identifies S1 and S2 heart sounds.			
8. Correctly obtains pulse deficit (apical rate minus radial rate).			

Recommendation: Pass _____ Needs more practice _____

Student: _____   Date: _____

Instructor: _____   Date: _____

PROCEDURE CHECKLIST
Chapter 17: Measuring Blood Pressure

Check (✓) Yes or No

PROCEDURE STEPS	Yes	No	COMMENTS
1. If possible, positions patient sitting, feet on floor, legs uncrossed; alternatively, lying down.			
2. Measures BP after patient has been inactive for 5 min.			
3. Exposes arm (does not auscultate through clothing).			
4. Supports patient's arm at the level of the heart.			
5. Uses appropriately sized cuff. (The width of the bladder of a properly fitting cuff will cover approximately 2/3 of the length of the upper arm for an adult, and the entire upper arm for a child. Alternatively, the length of the bladder encircles 80% to 100% of the arm in adults.)			
6. Positions cuff correctly; wraps snugly.			
7. Palpates radial artery, closes sphygmomanometer valve, and inflates cuff to determine mm Hg at which radial artery can no longer be felt.			
8. Places stethoscope on brachial artery and continues to inflate cuff rapidly to 30 mm Hg above level previously determined by palpation.			
9. Ensures that stethoscope tubing is not touching anything.			
10. Releases pressure at 2–3 mm Hg/second.			
11. Reads mercury manometer at eye level			
12. Records at least systolic/diastolic (first and last sounds heard—e.g., 110/80). Records level of muffling, if possible.			
13. If necessary to remeasure, waits at least 2 minutes.			

Recommendation: Pass _____ Needs more practice _____

Student: _____ Date: _____

Instructor: _____ Date: _____

PROCEDURE CHECKLIST
Chapter 19: Assessing the Abdomen

Check (✓) Yes or No

PROCEDURE STEPS	Yes	No	COMMENTS
1. Has the client void prior to the exam.			
2. Positions the client supine with the knees slightly flexed.			
3. Examines abdomen in this order: inspection, auscultation, percussion, palpation.			
4. Inspects the abdomen for:			
a. Size, symmetry, and contour.			
b. Has client raise his head to check for bulges.			
c. If distention is present, measures girth at umbilicus with tape measure.			
d. Observes the condition of skin and skin color; lesions, scars, striae, superficial veins, and hair distribution.			
e. Notes abdominal movements.			
f. Notes position, contour, and color of the umbilicus.			
4. Auscultates the abdomen for bowel sounds, using diaphragm of stethoscope.			
a. Listens for 5 min. before concluding that bowel sounds are absent.			
b. Uses stethoscope bell to listen for bruits.			
c. Listens for bruits over aorta and renal, femoral, and iliac arteries.			
5a. Uses indirect percussion to assess at multiple sites in all four quadrants.			
5b. Estimates size of liver, spleen, and bladder.			
6. Uses fist or blunt percussion to percuss the costovertebral angle for tenderness.			
7. Palpates abdomen:			
a. Begins with light palpation then uses deep palpation to palpate organs and masses.			
b. For light palpation, presses down 1–2 cm in a rotating motion. Identifies surface characteristics, tenderness, muscular resistance, and turgor.			

PROCEDURE STEPS	Yes	No	COMMENTS
8. Palpates liver:			
a. Places right hand at the client's midclavicular line under and parallel to the costal margin.			
b. Places left hand under the client's back at the lower ribs and pressing upward.			
c. Asks client to inhale and deeply exhale while pressing in and up with the right fingers.			
9. Palpates spleen by:			
a. Stands at client's right side.			
b. Places left hand under costovertebral angle and pulls upward.			
c. Places right hand under the left costal margin.			
d. Asks client to exhale and presses hands inward to palpate spleen.			

Recommendation: Pass _____ Needs more practice _____

Student: _____ Date: _____

Instructor: _____ Date: _____

Check (✓) Yes or No

PROCEDURE STEPS	Yes	No	COMMENTS
1. Inspects the anus, noting condition of the skin and presence of lesions.			

2. Palpates the anus and rectum.
 	
    a. *For women*: Changes gloves to prevent cross-contamination. Inserts a lubricated index finger gently into the rectum. Palpates the rectal wall noting masses or tenderness.
    b. *For men*: Has the client bend over the exam table or turn on his left side if recumbent. Inserts a lubricated index finger gently into the rectum. Palpates the rectal wall noting masses or tenderness.			

3. Tests any stool on the gloved finger for occult blood. (For reference, go to Procedure Checklist Chapter 28: Testing Stoll for Occult Blood.)			

Recommendation: Pass _____ Needs more practice _____

Student: _____   Date: _____

Instructor: _____   Date: _____

PROCEDURE CHECKLIST
Chapter 19: Assessing the Breasts and Axillae

Check [✓] Yes or No

PROCEDURE STEPS	Yes	No	COMMENTS
1. Inspects the breasts, nipples, areola, and axillae for skin condition, size, shape, symmetry, and color. Notes hair distribution in axillae.			

2. Inspects with client in these positions:
  a. Sitting, arms at sides.
  b. Sitting, arms raised overhead.
  c. Sitting, hands pressed on the hips.
  d. Sitting and leaning forward.
  e. Supine with a pillow under the shoulder of the breast being examined.			

3. Compares breasts bilaterally.			
4. Inspects nipples for discharge; if present, obtains a culture.			

5. Uses fingerpads of the 3 middle fingers to palpate the breasts using the vertical strip method, pie wedge, or concentric circles.
 	
Vertical strip method:
  Starts at the sternal edge and palpates the breast in parallel lines until reaching the midaxillary line. Goes up one area and down the adjacent strip (like "mowing the grass").
 	
Pie wedge method:
  This method examines the breast in wedges. Moves from one wedge to the next.
 	
Concentric circles method:
  Starts in the outermost area of the breast at the 12 o'clock position. Moves clockwise in concentric, ever smaller, circles.			

5a. Does not remove fingers from skin surface while palpating; moves by sliding fingers along the skin.			

PROCEDURE STEPS	Yes	No	COMMENTS
6. Palpates the nipples and areola.			
a. Notes tissue elasticity and tenderness.			
b. Squeezes nipple gently between thumb and finger to check for discharge.			
c. If open lesion or nipple discharge is present, wears procedure gloves to palpate the breasts.			
7. Palpates axillae and clavicular lymph nodes.			
a. Patient sitting with arms at sides, or supine.			
b. Uses fingerpads and moves fingers in circular fashion.			
c. Palpates all nodes: central, anterior pectoral, lateral brachial, posterior subscapular, epitrochlear, infraclavicular, supraclavicular.			

Recommendation: Pass _____ Needs more practice _____

Student: _____   Date: _____

Instructor: _____   Date: _____

PROCEDURE CHECKLIST
Chapter 19: Assessing the Chest and Lungs

Check [✓] Yes or No

PROCEDURE STEPS	Yes	No	COMMENTS
1. Assesses respirations by counting the respiratory rate and observing the rhythm, depth, and symmetry of chest movement.			
2. Inspects the chest for AP: lateral diameter, costal angle, spinal deformity, respiratory effort, and skin condition.			
3. Palpates trachea with fingers and thumb.			
4. Palpates the chest. a. Palpates for tenderness, masses or crepitus. b. Places hands on chest wall: anterior, posterior, and lateral.			
5. Palpates chest excursion. a. Places hands at the base of the chest with fingers spread and thumbs about 2 inches (5 cm) apart (at the costal margin anteriorly and at the 8th to 10th rib posteriorly). b. Presses thumbs toward the spine to create a small skinfold between them. c. Has the client take a deep breath and feels for chest expansion.			
6. Palpates chest for tactile fremitus.			
7. Percusses chest. a. Percusses over intercostal spaces rather than over bones.			
b. Uses indirect method of percussion.			
c. Percusses anterior, posterior, and lateral.			
d. Compares right side to left side.			
8. Percusses diaphragmatic excursion			
a. Percusses diaphragm level on full expiration; marks level.			
b. Percusses diaphragm level on full inspiration; marks level.			
c. Measures distance between the two marks.			

PROCEDURE STEPS	Yes	No	COMMENTS

9. Auscultates the chest.
 	
   a. Using same pattern as for percussion.
   b. Using diaphragm of stethoscope.
   c. Has client take slow, deep breaths through his mouth while listening at each site through one full respiratory cycle.			

10. Auscultates for abnormal voice sounds if there is evidence of lung congestion. Correctly uses one of the following methods, following the same pattern as for auscultation:			
a. Assesses for bronchophony by having the client say "1, 2, 3" as nurse listens over the lung fields.			
b. Assesses for egophony by having client say "eee" while listening over the lung fields.			
c. Assesses for Whispered Pectoriloquy by having client whisper "1, 2, 3" while listening over the lung fields.			

Recommendation: Pass _____ Needs more practice _____

Student: _____ Date: _____

Instructor: _____ Date: _____

PROCEDURE CHECKLIST
Chapter 19: Assessing the Ears and Hearing

Check (✓) Yes or No

PROCEDURE STEPS	Yes	No	COMMENTS
1. Inspect the external ear for placement, size, shape, symmetry, drainage, lesions, and color and condition of skin.			
2. Palpate the external structures of the ear for condition of skin and tenderness.			
3. Using otoscope, inspects tympanic membrane and bony landmarks.			
a. Uses correct size speculum.			
b. Has patient tilt head to side not being examined.			
c. Looks for foreign object in canal before inserting scope.			
d. *For Adult*: Pulls helix up and back. *For Preschool Child*: Pulls helix down and back.			
e. Inserts speculum slowly, only into outer 1/3 of canal.			
f. Identifies location of cone of light and bony landmarks.			
g. Uses "puff" of air to test TM mobility.			
4. Tests gross hearing.			
a. Stands 1 to 2 feet behind the patient. Has the patient cover one ear as you whisper some words. Repeats on the other side. Has the patient repeat the words heard.			
b. Has the patient occlude one ear. Holds a ticking watch next to the patient's unobstructed ear. Slowly moves it away until the patient says he can hear the sound.			
5. Performs Weber test (places vibrating tuning fork on top of patient's head, identifying as positive if sound not heard equally in both ears).			

PROCEDURE STEPS	Yes	No	COMMENTS

6. Performs Rinne test if Weber is positive.
   a. Strikes a tuning fork on the table. While it is still vibrating, places it on the patient's mastoid process.
   b. Measures the time in seconds that the patient hears the vibration.
   c. Moves the tuning fork to 1 inch (2.5 cm) in front of the ear and measure the time until the patient can no longer hear the vibration.
   d. Compares AC and BC times.			

7. Performs Romberg test: Has client stand with feet together, hands at side with eyes opened and then with eyes closed. Notes ability to maintain balance. Identifies swaying as positive Romberg.			
8. Compares bilaterally throughout examination.			

Recommendation: Pass _____ Needs more practice _____

Student: _____   Date: _____

Instructor: _____   Date: _____

Check (✓) Yes or No

PROCEDURE STEPS	Yes	No	COMMENTS
1. Assesses distance vision using a Snellen chart.			
a. Chooses correct chart for age and literacy.			
b. Allows client to wear corrective lenses for test.			
c. Has patient stand 20 ft from chart and cover one eye at a time.			
d. Tests eyes singly and then together.			
e. Records findings correctly.			
2. Tests near vision by measuring the ability to read newsprint at a distance of 14 inches (35 cm). Correctly identifies hyperopia or presbyopia if present.			
3. Tests color vision by using color plates or the color bars on the Snellen chart.			
4. Assesses peripheral vision by determining when an object comes into sight.			
a. Seats client 2 to 3 feet from nurse			
b. Has client cover one eye and gaze straight ahead.			
c. Begins well outside normal peripheral vision and brings object to the center of the visual fields.			
d. Repeats in all 4 visual fields, clockwise.			
5. Assesses EOMs by examining: a. for parallel alignment. b. the corneal light reflex. c. the ability to move through the six cardinal gaze positions. d. the cover/uncover test.			
6. Inspects external structures: a. Color and alignment of eyes.			
b. Eyelids: notes any lesions, edema, or lid lag.			
c. Symmetry and distribution of eyelashes.			
d. Lacrimal ducts and glands, checks for edema, and drainage.			
e. Notes color, moisture, and contour of conjunctiva.			
f. Inspects both palpebral and bulbar conjunctiva.			
g. Sclera: Notes color and presence of lesions.			
h. Inspects cornea and lens with penlight; notes color and lesions.			
i. Tests the corneal reflex with a cotton wisp.			

PROCEDURE STEPS	Yes	No	COMMENTS
j. Notes color, size, shape, and symmetry of iris and pupils.			
k. Checks pupil reaction for direct and consensual response.			
l. Assesses pupil accommodation by having the patient focus on an approaching object.			
m. Inspects anterior chamber with penlight, for color, size, shape, and symmetry.			
7. Palpates the external eye structures for tenderness and discharge; palpates globes and lacrimal glands and ducts.			
8. Assesses the internal structures via ophthalmoscopy. Darkens the room.			
a. Stands about 1 foot from the patient at a 15 degree lateral angle.			
b. Dials the lens wheel to zero with index finger.			
c. Holds ophthalmoscope to own brow.			
d. Has the patient look straight ahead while shining the light on one pupil to identify the red light reflex.			
e. Once the red light reflex is identified, moves in closer to within a few inches of the eye and observes the internal structures of the eye. Adjusts the lens wheel to focus as needed.			
f. Uses right eye to examine the patient's right eye, and left eye to examine the patient's left eye.			

Recommendation: Pass _____ Needs more practice _____

Student: _____   Date: _____

Instructor: _____   Date: _____

PROCEDURE CHECKLIST
Chapter 19: Assessing the Female Genitourinary System

Check (✓) Yes or No

PROCEDURE STEPS	Yes	No	COMMENTS
1. Instructs client to disrobe to expose the pelvic area.			
2. Positions patient in lithotomy or Sims position, providing support as needed.			
3. Inspects external genitalia.			
a. Notes distribution and condition of pubic hair.			
b. Inspects mons, pubis, and labia for color, lesions, and discharge.			
4. Wearing gloves, uses thumb and index finger to separate the labia and expose the clitoris; observes for size and position.			
5. With labia separated, observes urethral meatus and vaginal introitus for color, size, and presence of discharge or lesions. Then asks client to bear down while observing the introitus for bulging or discomfort.			
6. Palpates Bartholin's and Skene's glands.			
a. Lubricates gloved middle and index fingers of dominant hand with water soluble lubricant.			
b. Palpates Bartholin's gland by inserting fingers into the introitus and palpating the lower portion of the labia bilaterally between thumb and fingers.			
c. Palpates Skene's glands by then rotating the internal fingers upward and palpating the labia bilaterally.			
d. Milks the urethra by applying pressure with index finger on the anterior vaginal wall; cultures any discharge.			
7. Assesses vaginal and pelvic muscle tone by inserting 2 gloved fingers into the vagina and asking the woman to constrict her vaginal muscles, and then to bear down as if she is having a bowel movement.			
8. Palpates lymph nodes in the groin area and the vertical chain over the inner aspect of the thigh.			

Recommendation: Pass _____ Needs more practice _____

Student: _____   Date: _____

Instructor: _____   Date: _____

PROCEDURE CHECKLIST
Chapter 19: Assessing the Hair

Check (✓) Yes or No

PROCEDURE STEPS	Yes	No	COMMENTS
1. Assesses both scalp hair and body hair.			
2. Inspects and palpates scalp; notes mobility, tenderness, and lesions.			
3. Assesses hair color, quantity, and distribution; condition of scalp; and presence of lesions or pediculosis.			
4. Palpates hair texture.			

Recommendation: Pass _____ Needs more practice _____

Student: _____   Date: _____

Instructor: _____   Date: _____

PROCEDURE CHECKLIST
Chapter 19: Assessing the Head and Face

Check (✓) Yes or No

PROCEDURE STEPS	Yes	No	COMMENTS
1. Compares side to side throughout the exam.			
2. Inspects head for size, shape, symmetry, and position.			
3. Inspects face for expression and symmetry.			
4. Palpates head for masses, tenderness, and scalp mobility.			
5. Palpates face for symmetry, tenderness, muscle tone and TMJ function.			

Recommendation: Pass _____ Needs more practice _____

Student: _____   Date: _____

Instructor: _____   Date: _____

Check (✓) Yes or No

PROCEDURE STEPS	Yes	No	COMMENTS
1. Inspects the neck and chest.			
a. Positions patient supine.			
b. Observes carotid arteries.			
2. Assesses jugular flow by compressing jugular vein below the jaw and observing jugular wave.			
3. Assesses jugular filling by compressing jugular vein above the clavicle and observing for disappearance of jugular wave.			

4. Measures jugular venous pressure (JVP).
  a. Elevates the head of the bed to a 45° angle.
  b. Identifies the highest point of visible internal jugular filling.
  c. Places a ruler vertically at the sternal angle (*where the clavicles meet*).
  d. Places another ruler horizontally at the highest point of the venous wave.
  e. Measures the distance in centimeters vertically from the chest wall.			

5. Places patient supine with tangential lighting to inspect precordium for pulsations.			
6. Palpates the carotid arteries.			
a. Palpates each side separately.			
b. Avoids massaging the artery.			
c. Notes rate, rhythm, amplitude, and symmetry of pulse.			
d. Notes contour, symmetry, and elasticity of the arteries; notes any thrills.			
7. Palpates the precordium.			
a. Has patient sit up and lean forward; if lying down, turns patient to the left side.			
b. Palpates: apex, left lateral sternal border, epigastric area, base left, and base right.			
8. Works from patient's right side to auscultate, if possible.			
9. Auscultates the carotids: uses bell of stethoscope, has patient hold his breath while listening.			

PROCEDURE STEPS	Yes	No	COMMENTS
10. Auscultates jugular veins: uses bell of stethoscope, has patient hold his breath while listening.			
11. Auscultates the precordium: a. Identifies S1, S2, S3, and S4 sounds. b. Listens for murmurs. c. Listens with both bell and diaphragm at all four locations.			
d. Listens at: base right (aortic valve), base left (pulmonic valve), apex (mitral valve), and left lateral sternal border (tricuspid valve).			
12. If murmur is heard, identifies variables affecting (e.g., location, quality, pitch, intensity, timing, duration, configuration, radiation, and respiratory variation) and compares with previous findings. Refers to primary care if murmur is a new finding.			
13. Inspects the periphery for color, temperature, and edema.			
14. Palpates the peripheral pulses: radial, brachial, femoral, popliteal, dorsalis pedis, and posterior tibial.			
a. Uses distal pads of 2nd and 3rd fingers to firmly palpate pulses.			
b. Palpates firmly but does not occlude artery.			
c. Assesses pulses for rate, rhythm, equality, amplitude, and elasticity.			
d. Describes pulse amplitude on a scale of 0 to 4: 0 = absent, not palpable 1 = diminished, barely palpable 2 = normal, expected 3 = full, increased 4 = bounding			
15. Inspects the venous system. If a client has varicosities, assess for valve competence with the manual compression test.			

Recommendation: Pass _____ Needs more practice _____

Student: _____   Date: _____

Instructor: _____   Date: _____

PROCEDURE CHECKLIST
Chapter 19: Assessing the Male Genitourinary System

Check (✓) Yes or No

PROCEDURE STEPS	Yes	No	COMMENTS
1. Instructs client to empty his bladder and undress to expose the groin area.			
2. Positions patient standing and sits at eye level to the genitalia; or positions patient supine with legs slightly apart.			
3. Inspects external genitalia.			
a. Notes distribution and condition of pubic hair.			
b. Inspects penis, noting condition of skin, presence or absence of foreskin, position of urethral meatus, and any lesions or discharge.			
c. Observes the scrotum for: skin condition, size, position, and symmetry.			
d. Inspects inguinal areas for swelling or bulges.			
4. Palpates penis.			
a. Uses thumb and fingers of gloved hand.			
b. Notes consistency, tenderness, masses, or nodules.			
c. Retracts foreskin if present.			
5. Palpates scrotum, testes, and epididymis.			
a. Uses thumb and fingers of gloved hand. Notes size, shape, consistency, mobility, masses, nodules, or tenderness.			
b. Transilluminates any lumps, nodules, or edematous areas by shinning a pen light over the area in a darkened room.			
6. Palpates for inguinal hernias with a gloved hand. Has the patient hold his penis to one side. Places index finger in the client's scrotal sac above the testicle and invaginates the skin. Follows the spermatic cord until reaching a slitlike opening (Hesselbach's triangle). Asks the client to cough or bear down while feeling for bulges.			
7. Palpates for femoral hernias by palpating below the femoral artery while having the client cough or bear down.			
8. Palpates the lymph nodes in the groin area and the vertical chain over the inner aspect of the thigh.			

Recommendation: Pass _____ Needs more practice _____

Student: _____   Date: _____

Instructor: _____   Date: _____

PROCEDURE CHECKLIST
Chapter 19: Assessing the Mouth and Oropharynx

Check (✓) Yes or No

PROCEDURE STEPS	Yes	No	COMMENTS
1. Inspects mouth externally. Notes the placement, color, and condition of lips. Asks client to purse the lips.			
2. Notes color and condition of oral mucosa and gums: a. Inspects inside lower lip.			
b. Uses tongue depressor and penlight to inspect buccal mucosa, and Stensen's ducts.			
c. Palpates inside each cheek.			
d. Inspects gums for color, bleeding, edema, retraction, and lesions.			
e. Palpates gums for firmness.			
3. Inspects teeth for color, condition, and occlusion.			
4. If client wears dentures, asks her to remove them; inspects for condition and fit.			
5. Inspects tongue and floor of the mouth. a. Asks client to stick out his tongue. Examines upper surface for color, texture, position, and mobility.			
b. Has client place tip of tongue on roof of his mouth; uses penlight to inspect underside of tongue, frenulum, floor of mouth, and submaxillary glands.			
c. Using tongue blade or gloved finger, moves tongue aside and examines lateral aspects of tongue and floor of mouth.			
d. Palpates tongue and floor or mouth, stabilizing the tongue by grasping with a gauze pad.			
6. Inspects the oropharynx (hard/soft palate, tonsils and uvula); notes color, shape, texture, and condition.			
a. Has the client tilt his head back and open his mouth as widely as possible. Depresses the tongue with a tongue blade and shines a penlight on the areas to be inspected.			
b. To inspect the uvula, asks the client to say "ah" and watches the uvula as the soft palate rises.			
c. Inspects the oropharynx by depressing one side of the tongue at a time, about halfway back on the tongue.			
d. Notes the size and color of the tonsils; notes any discharge.			
7. Tests the gag reflex by touching the back of the soft palate with a tongue blade.			

PROCEDURE STEPS	Yes	No	COMMENTS

Recommendation: Pass _____ Needs more practice _____

Student: _____   Date: _____

Instructor: _____   Date: _____

PROCEDURE CHECKLIST
Chapter 19: Assessing the Musculoskeletal System

Check (✓) Yes or No

PROCEDURE STEPS	Yes	No	COMMENTS
1. Compares bilaterally during assessment.			
2. Assesses posture, body alignment, and symmetry.			

3. Assesses spinal curvature:
    a. Standing erect.
    b. Bending forward at waist, arms hanging free at sides.			

4. Examines gait by observing client walking; notes:
    a. Base of support (distance between the feet).
    b. Stride length (distance between each step).
    c. Phases of the gait.			

5. Assesses balance through:
    a. Tandem walking.
    b. Heel and toe walking.
    c. Deep knee bends.
    d. Hopping.
    e. Romberg test (feet together, eyes open; then eyes closed).			

6. Assesses coordination:
    a. Assesses with client seated.
    b. Tests finger-thumb opposition.
    c. Tests rapid alternating movements by having client alternate supination and pronation of the hands.
    d. Tests rhythmic toe-tapping, one side at a time.
    e. Has client run heel of one foot down the shin of the other leg; repeats on opposite side.			

7. Tests the accuracy of movements by having the client touch his finger to his nose with his eyes closed.			
8. Measures arm length from acromion process to the tip of the middle finger.			
9. Measures leg length from the anterior superior iliac crest to the medial malleolus.			
10. Measures circumference of forearms, upper arms, thighs, and calves.			
11. Inspects symmetry and shape of muscles and joints.			
12. Notes surgical scars indicating joint surgeries.			
13. Tests active ROM by asking client to move each of the following joints: temporomandibular, neck, thoracic and lumbar spine; shoulder, upper arm and elbow; wrist, hands, and fingers; hip, knee, ankles, and feet.			
14. Checks for the following joint movements:			

PROCEDURE STEPS		Yes	No	COMMENTS
a. Temporo-mandibular	Able to flex, extend, move side-to-side, protrude, and retract the jaw.			
b. Neck	Flexes, extends, hyperextends, bends laterally, and rotates side-to-side.			
c. Thoracic and lumbar spine	Able to bend at the waist, stand upright, hyperextend (bend backward), bend laterally, and rotate side-to-side.			
d. Shoulder	Able to move the arm forward and backward, abduct, adduct, and rotate internally and externally.			
e. Upper arm and elbow	Able to bend, extend, supinate, and pronate the elbow.			
f. Wrist	Flexes, extends, hyperextends, and moves side-to-side.			
g. Hands and fingers	Able to spread the fingers (abduct), bring them together (adduct), make a fist (flex), extend the hand (extend), bend fingers back (hyperextend), and bring thumb to index finger (palmar adduction).			
h. Hip	Able to extend the leg straight, flex the knee to the chest, abduct and adduct the leg, rotate the hip internally and externally, and hyperextend the leg.			
i. Knee	Able to flex and extend the knee.			
j. Ankles and feet	Able to dorsiflex, plantar flex, evert, invert, abduct, and adduct the feet and ankles.			
15. Assesses muscle strength by having the client perform ROM against resistance.				
16. Rates muscle strength correctly using the following rating scale:				

Rating	Criteria	Classification
5	Active motion against full resistance	Normal
4	Active motion against some resistance	Slight weakness
3	Active motion against gravity	Weakness
2	Passive ROM	Poor ROM
1	Slight flicker of contraction	Severe weakness
0	No muscular contraction	Paralysis

Recommendation: Pass _____ Needs more practice _____

Student: _____ Date: _____

Instructor: _____ Date: _____

PROCEDURE CHECKLIST
Chapter 19: Assessing the Nails

Check (✓) Yes or No

PROCEDURE STEPS	Yes	No	COMMENTS
1. Compares bilaterally throughout exam.			
2. Inspects nails for color, condition, and shape.			
3. Palpates the texture of the nails.			
4. Correctly assesses capillary refill by pressing on the nails and releasing.			
5. Examines nails on both hands and feet; or states he will defer examination of the toenails until the assessment of peripheral circulation.			

Recommendation: Pass _____ Needs more practice _____

Student: _____   Date: _____

Instructor: _____   Date: _____

PROCEDURE CHECKLIST
Chapter 19: Assessing the Neck

Check (✓) Yes or No

PROCEDURE STEPS	Yes	No	COMMENTS
1. Inspects the neck in neutral and hyperextended position, and while patient swallows water.			
2. Notes symmetry, range of motion (ROM), and condition of skin.			
3. Palpates the cervical lymph nodes. 　a. Uses light palpation with one or two fingerpads, in a circular movement.			
b. Palpates all nodes: pre-auricular, posterior auricular, tonsillar, submandibular, submental, occipital, superficial cervical, deep cervical, posterior cervical, and supraclavicular.			
c. Notes the size, shape, symmetry, consistency, mobility, tenderness, and temperature of any palpable nodes.			
4. Palpates the thyroid, using correct technique. **To use the posterior approach:** 　a. Stands behind the client and asks him to flex his neck slightly forward and to the left. 　b. Positions thumbs on the nape of the client's neck. 　c. Using the fingers of the left hand, locates the cricoid cartilage. Pushes the trachea slightly to the left with the right hand while palpating just below the cricoid and between the trachea and sternocleidomastoid muscle. Asks client to swallow (gives small sips of water if necessary) and feels for the thyroid gland as it rises up. 　d. Reverses and repeats the same steps to palpate the right thyroid lobe (uses fingers of left hand to displace the trachea to the right while using the fingers of the right hand to palpate the thyroid to the right of the trachea).			

PROCEDURE STEPS	Yes	No	COMMENTS
To use the anterior approach: a. Stands in front of the client and asks him to flex his neck slightly forward and in the direction the nurse intends to palpate. b. Places hands on the neck and applies gentle pressure to one side of the trachea while palpating the opposite side of the neck for the thyroid as the client swallows. c. Reverses and repeats the same steps on the opposite side.			
5. If thyroid is enlarged, or there is a mass, follows up with auscultation of the gland.			

Recommendation: Pass _____ Needs more practice _____

Student: _____   Date: _____

Instructor: _____   Date: _____

Check (✓) Yes or No

PROCEDURE STEPS	Yes	No	COMMENTS
1. Compares right and left sides throughout examination.			
2. Inspects the external nose. a. Notes the position, shape, and size; discharge and flaring.			
3. Checks for patency of the nasal passages. a. Asks the client to close his mouth, hold one naris closed, and breathe through the other naris. Repeats with opposite naris.			
4. Inspects the internal structures. a. Holds speculum in right hand to inspect left nostril; in left hand to inspect right nostril.			
b. Tilts the client's head back to facilitate speculum insertion and visualization.			
c. Braces index finger against the client's nose as inserting the speculum..			
d. Inserts the speculum about 1 cm into the naris; opens as much as possible.			
e. Uses the other hand to position client's head and hold penlight.			
f. Observes the nasal mucosa for color, edema, lesions, and discharge.			
g. Inspects the septum for position and intactness.			
h. *Infants and children*—Does not use a speculum to examine internal structures. Pushes the tip of the nose upward with thumb and directs a penlight into the nares.			
5. Transilluminates the frontal and maxillary sinuses. a. Darkens the room.			
b. *Frontal sinuses*: Shines a penlight or the otoscope with speculum below eyebrow on each side.			
c. *Maxillary sinuses*: Places the light source below the eyes and above the cheeks. Looks for a glow of red light at the roof of the mouth through the client's open mouth.			
6. Palpates the external structures.			
7. Palpates the frontal and maxillary sinuses.			

Recommendation: Pass _____ Needs more practice _____

Student: _____   Date: _____

Instructor: _____   Date: _____

PROCEDURE CHECKLIST
Chapter 19: Assessing the Sensory-Neurological System

Check (✓) Yes or No

PROCEDURE STEPS	Yes	No	COMMENTS
1. Assesses behavior, noting facial expression, posture, affect, and grooming.			
2. Determines level of arousal using, as needed, and in this order: verbal stimuli, tactile stimuli, painful stimuli.			
3. Correctly describes altered levels of arousal using the Glasgow Coma Scale.			
4. Determines level of orientation.			
a. Checks orientation to time.			
b. Checks orientation to place.			
c. Checks orientation to person.			
5. Assesses immediate, recent, and remote memory. Uses correct method to assess each type of memory: a. Immediate memory (asks client to repeat a series of numbers, beginning with a series of three). Then repeats test, asking client to repeat numbers in reverse order.			
b. Recent memory (names 3 items and asks client to recall them later in the exam; or asks "How did you get to the hospital?" and so forth).			
c. Remote memory (asks birth date, for example).			
6. Assesses mathematical and calculative skills, beginning with simplest problem and progressing to more difficult.			
a. Considers the person's language, education, and culture in deciding whether this test is appropriate for him.			
b. Uses the following tests, as appropriate: 1) Has the client solve a simple mathematical problem, such as 3 +3. 2) If client is able to solve that problem, presents a more complex example, such as: If you have $3.00 and you buy an item for $2.00, how much money will you have left? 3) To assess both calculation skills and attention span, asks the client to count backward from 100. 4) A more difficult test is to have the client perform *serial threes* or *serial sevens*. Asks him to begin at 100 and keep subtracting 3 (or 7).			

PROCEDURE STEPS	Yes	No	COMMENTS
7. Assesses general knowledge by asking the client how many days in the week or months in the year.			
8. Evaluates thought processes throughout the exam. Assesses attention span, logic of speech, ability to stay focused, and appropriateness of responses.			
9. Assesses abstract thinking, for example, by asking the client to interpret a proverb, such as "A penny saved is a penny earned."			
10. Assesses judgment by asking the client to respond to a hypothetical situation, such as "If you were walking down the street and saw smoke and flame coming from a house, what would you do?"			
11. Assesses communication ability.			
a. During the exam, notes the rate, flow, choice of vocabulary, and enunciation in client's speech.			
b. Tests spontaneous speech: Shows client a picture and has him describe it.			
c. Tests motor speech by having the client say "do, re, mi, fa, so, la, ti, do."			
d. Tests automatic speech by having the client recite the days of the week.			
e. Tests sound recognition by having the client identify a familiar sound, such as clapping hands.			
f. Tests auditory-verbal comprehension by asking the client to follow simple directions (e.g., point to your nose, rub your left elbow).			
g. Tests visual recognition by pointing to objects and asking the client to identify them.			
h. Tests visual-verbal comprehension by having the client read a sentence and explain its meaning.			
i. Tests writing by having the client write his name and address.			
j. Tests copying figures by having the client copy a circle, x, square, triangle and star.			
12. CN I–checks patency of nostrils, checks one nostril at a time for client's ability to identify the smell of common substances.			
13. CN II–tests visual acuity and visual fields; performs fundoscopic exam.			

PROCEDURE STEPS	Yes	No	COMMENTS
14. CN III, IV, and VI– a. Tests EOMs by having the client move the eyes through the 6 cardinal fields of gaze with the head held steady. b. Tests pupillary reaction to light and accommodation.			
15. CN V, motor function–has client move his jaw from side to side, clenching his jaw, and biting down on a tongue blade.			
16. CN V, sensory function–has the client close his eyes and identify when nurse is touching his face at the forehead, cheeks, and chin bilaterally—first with the finger and then with a toothpick.			
17. Tests corneal reflex by touching the cornea with a wisp of cotton or puffing air from a syringe over the cornea.			
18. CN VII, motor function–has the client make faces, such as smile, frown or whistle.			
19. CN VII, taste–tests taste on the anterior portion of the tongue by placing sweet (sugar), salty (salt), or sour (lemon) substance on tip of tongue.			
20. CN VIII–Uses: a. Watch-tick test for hearing. b. Weber and Rinne tests for air and bone conduction. c. Romberg test for balance (if not already done).			
21. CN IX and X–observes ability to talk, swallow, and cough.			
22. CN IX and X, motor function–asks client to say "ah" while depressing tongue with a tongue blade and observing the soft palate and uvula to rise.			
23. CN IX and X, sensory function–touches back of pharynx with tongue blade to induce a gag reflex.			
24. CN IX and X, taste (sweet, salty, sour)–tests on posterior portion of tongue.			
25. CN XI (if not assessed with musculoskeletal exam): a. Places hands on client's shoulders and has client shrug his shoulders against resistance. b. Has client turn his head from side to side against resistance.			
26. CN XII–has the client: a. Say "d, l, n, t." b. Protrude the tongue and move it from side to side.			
27. When testing superficial sensations:			

PROCEDURE STEPS	Yes	No	COMMENTS
a. Begins with the most peripheral part of the limb.			
b. If client does not perceive the touch, determines boundaries by testing at about every inch (2.5 cm); sketches the area of sensory loss.			
c. Waits 2 seconds before moving to a new site.			
d. Tests first with wisp of cotton, then tests for pain with toothpick or sterile needle (first the dull, then the sharp end).			
e. Alternates dull and sharp ends when moving from spot to spot.			
f. Tests temperature sensation if pain perception is abnormal.			
28. Tests deep vibratory sensation by placing a vibrating tuning fork on a metatarsal joint and distal interphalangeal joint and having the patient identify when the vibration is felt and when it stops.			
29. Tests deep kinesthetic sensation (position sense) by holding the client's finger or toe on the sides and moving it up or down. Instructs client to keep his eyes closed and identify the direction of the movement.			
30. Performs all discriminatory sensation tests: stereognosis, graphesthesia, 2-point discrimination, point localization, and sensory extinction.			
31. Uses correct procedure to test discriminatory sensation tests:			
a. Assesses stereognosis by placing a familiar object (e.g., a coin or a button) in the palm of the client's hand and having him identify it.			
b. Assesses graphesthesia by drawing a number or letter in the palm of patient's hand and having the patient identify what was drawn.			
c. Tests 2-point discrimination with toothpicks. Has the patient close his eyes. Touches him on the finger with 2 separate toothpicks simultaneously. Gradually moves the points together and has the patient say "one" or "two" each time the toothpicks are moved. Documents distance and location at which he can no longer feel 2 separate points.			
d. Tests point localization by having the patient close his eyes while the nurse touches him. Have him point to the area touched. Repeat on both sides and upper and lower extremities.			

PROCEDURE STEPS	Yes	No	COMMENTS
e. Tests sensory extinction by simultaneously touching the patient on both sides (e.g., on both hands, both knees, both arms). Has the patient identify where he was touched.			
32. Tests each of the following deep tendon reflexes: biceps, triceps, brachioradialis, patellar, and Achilles.			
33. Uses correct procedure to test each reflex: a. Biceps reflex (spinal cord level C–5 and C–6). Rests the patient's elbow in nondominant hand, with thumb over the biceps tendon. Strikes the percussion hammer to own thumb.			
b. Triceps reflex (spinal cord level C–7 and C–8). Abducts patient's arm at the shoulder and flexes it at the elbow. Supports the upper arm with nondominant hand, letting the forearm hang loosely. Strikes the triceps tendon about 1–2 inches (2.5 to 5 cm) above the olecranon process.			
c. Brachioradialis reflex (spinal cord level C–3 and C–6). Rests patient's arm on patient's leg. Strikes with the percussion hammer 1–2 inches (2.5 to 5 cm) above the bony prominence of the wrist on the thumb side.			
d. Patellar reflex (spinal cord level L–2, L–3, and L–4). Has patient sit with legs dangling. Strikes the tendon directly below the patella.			
e. Achilles reflex (spinal cord level S–1, S–2). Has the patient lie supine or sit with the legs dangling. Holds the patient's foot slightly dorsiflexed and strikes the Achilles tendon about 2 inches (5 cm) above the heel with the percussion hammer.			
34. Uses the following scale to grade reflexes: 0 No response detected +1 Diminished response +2 Response normal +3 Response somewhat stronger than normal +4 Response hyperactive with clonus			
35. Tests plantar superficial reflex with thumbnail or pointed object. Strokes sole of foot in an arc from the lateral heel to medially across the ball of the foot.			

Recommendation: Pass _____ Needs more practice _____

Student: _____   Date: _____

Instructor: _____   Date: _____

Check (✓) Yes or No

PROCEDURE STEPS	Yes	No	COMMENTS
1. Uses inspection, palpation, and olfaction.			
2. Assesses both exposed and unexposed areas.			
3. Compares side to side throughout exam.			
4. Inspects skin color.			
5. Notes unusual odors.			
6. Inspects and palpates lesions.			
7. For identified lesions, describes size, shape, color, distribution, texture, surface relationship, exudates, tenderness, or pain.			
8. Uses ABCDE method to evaluate lesions that may need referral due to potential malignancy.			
9. Palpates skin temperature with dorsal aspect of hand or fingers.			
10. Palpates skin turgor by gently pulling up skin and noting its return.			
11. Palpates skin texture, moisture, and hydration.			
12. Inspects for edema. Notes location, degree, and type if present.			
13. Considers culture/ethnicity, gender, and developmental stage of client in interpreting data.			

Recommendation: Pass _____ Needs more practice _____

Student: _____   Date: _____

Instructor: _____   Date: _____

PROCEDURE CHECKLIST
Chapter 19: Performing the General Survey

Check (✓) Yes or No

PROCEDURE STEPS	Yes	No	COMMENTS
1. Observes for signs of distress; alters approach if patient is distressed.			
2. Observes apparent age, gender, and race.			
3. Notes facial characteristics, symmetry of features, expression, and condition and color of skin.			
4. Notes body type and posture.			
5. Greets patient with handshake to assess muscle strength (if culturally appropriate).			
6. Observes gait and any abnormal movements (or ability to move about in bed).			
7. Listens to speech pattern, pace, quality, tone, vocabulary, and sentence structure.			
8. Obtains interpreter if there is a language barrier.			
9. Assesses general mental state and affect.			
10. Observes dress, grooming, and hygiene.			
11. Measures vital signs.			
12. Measures height and weight. 　　a. *Adults*: Calculates BMI from height and weight measurement.			
b. *Infants and children < 2 years*: Height—positions supine with knees extended; also measures head circumference.			
c. *Infants*: Weighs without clothing; 　　d. *Older children*: Weighs in underwear.			
13. For children, plots height and weight on growth chart and evaluates trends.			

Recommendation: Pass _____ Needs more practice _____

Student: _____   Date: _____

Instructor: _____   Date: _____

PROCEDURE CHECKLIST
Chapter 20: Applying Sterile Gloves (Open Method)

Check (✓) Yes or No

PROCEDURE STEPS	Yes	No	COMMENTS
1. Opens outer wrapper and places glove package on a clean dry surface.			
2. Opens inner package so that glove cuffs are nearest to the nurse.			
3. Fully opens the package flaps so they do not fold back over and contaminate the gloves.			
4. Takes care to not touch anything else on the sterile field, with nondominant hand grasps the inner surface of the glove for the dominant hand and lifts up and away from the table.			
5. Slides dominant hand into the glove, keeping hand and fingers above the waist and away from the body.			
6. Slides gloved fingers under the cuff of the glove for the nondominant hand.			
7. Lifts the glove up and away from the table and away from the body.			
8. Slides nondominant hand into the glove, avoiding contact with the gloved hand.			
9. Adjusts both gloves to fit the fingers and so that there is no excess at the fingertips.			
10. Keeps hands between shoulder and waist level.			

Recommendation: Pass _____ Needs more practice _____

Student: _____   Date: _____

Instructor: _____   Date: _____

PROCEDURE CHECKLIST
Chapter 20: Donning Personal Protective Equipment (PPE)

Check (✓) Yes or No

PROCEDURE STEPS	Yes	No	COMMENTS
1. Assesses need for personal protective equipment. *Gloves*: When the nurse may be exposed to potentially infectious secretions or materials. *Gowns*: When the nurse's uniform may get exposed to potentially infectious secretions. *Face mask*: When splashing may occur and potentially contaminate the nurse's mouth or nose. *Face shield or eye goggles*: When splashing may occur and potentially contaminate the nurse's eyes.			
2. Determines availability of appropriate personal protective equipment.			
3. Picks up gown by shoulders; allows to fall open without touching any contaminated surface.			
4. Slips arms into the sleeves; fastens ties at the neck.			
5. If gown does not completely cover clothing, wears two gowns. Places the first gown on with the opening in the front and then places the second gown over the first with the opening in the back.			
6. Identifies the top edge of the mask by locating the thin metal strip that goes over the bridge of the nose.			
7. Picks up mask with the top ties or ear loops.			
8. Places metal strip over bridge of nose and ties upper ties or slips loops around ears.			
9. Places lower edge of mask below chin and ties lower ties.			
10. Presses metal strip so it conforms to the bridge of the nose.			
11. Dons face shield by placing shield over eyes, adjusting metal strip over bridge of nose, and tucking the lower edge below the chin. Secures straps behind head.			
12. Dons safety glasses or goggles by setting them over the top edge of the face mask.			
13. Selects appropriate size.			
14. If wearing a gown, makes sure that the glove cuff extends over the cuff of the gown.			
15. If there is not complete coverage, tapes the glove cuff to the gown.			

PROCEDURE STEPS	Yes	No	COMMENTS

Recommendation: Pass _____ Needs more practice _____

Student: _____   Date: _____

Instructor: _____   Date: _____

PROCEDURE CHECKLIST
Chapter 20: Donning Sterile Gown and Gloves (Closed Method)

Check (✓) Yes or No

PROCEDURE STEPS	Yes	No	COMMENTS
1. Grasps gown at the neckline, allows it to fall open while stepping back from the table.			
2. Does not allow gown to touch any nonsterile surface.			
3. Slides both arms into the sleeves without extending hands through the cuffs.			
4. Keeps the sleeves of the gown above waist level.			
5. Has a coworker pull up gown shoulders and tie neck tie (coworker touches only inside of gown).			
6. Opens the sterile glove wrapper, keeping fingers inside the sleeve of the gown.			
7. Keeping hands inside gown sleeves, grasps cuff of the glove for the dominant hand.			
8. Lays glove on forearm of the dominant hand, with the palm of the glove facing down, glove fingers pointed toward elbow, and glove thumb positioned on thumb side of dominant hand			
9. Grasps the inside glove cuff with dominant hand through the gown, being careful to keep fingers inside the gown.			
10. With nondominant hand encased in the gown sleeve, pulls the dominant-hand glove cuff over the cuff of the gown.			
11. Grasping sleeve of gown (nondominant hand) and the cuff of the dominant-hand glove, pulls the glove onto the dominant hand.			
12. Places second glove on the forearm of nondominant hand with the palm of the glove down, fingers pointed toward the elbow and glove thumb on thumb-side of nondominant hand.			
13. Grasps the inside glove cuff with nondominant hand through the gown, being careful to keep fingers inside the gown.			
14. With dominant hand, pulls the glove cuff over the cuff of the gown.			

PROCEDURE STEPS	Yes	No	COMMENTS
15. Grasps the sleeve of the gown and the cuff of the glove and pulls the glove onto the nondominant hand.			
16. Adjusts the fingers in both gloves.			
17. Grasps the waist tie on the gown and hands the tie to the circulating nurse or coworker who is wearing a hair cover and mask. Coworker grabs the tie with sterile forceps. Makes a 3/4 turn and receives the tie from coworker.			
18. Secures the waist tie.			

Recommendation: Pass _____ Needs more practice _____

Student: _____   Date: _____

Instructor: _____   Date: _____

PROCEDURE CHECKLIST
Chapter 20: Hand Washing

Check (✓) Yes or No

PROCEDURE STEPS	Yes	No	COMMENTS
1. Pushes up sleeves; removes jewelry and watches.			
2. Adjusts water temperature to warm.			
3. Wets hands and wrists under running water, keeping hands lower than wrists and forearms.			
4. Avoids splashing water onto clothing.			
5. Avoids touching inside of the sink.			
6. Applies 3 to 5 mL liquid soap.			
7. Rubs soap over all surfaces of hands.			
8. Rubs hands vigorously together for at least 15 seconds.			
9. Lathers all surfaces of the hands and fingers.			
10. Cleans under fingernails, if nails are dirty.			
11. Rinses thoroughly, keeping hands lower than forearms.			
12. Dries hands thoroughly: moves from fingers up forearms; blots with paper towel.			
13. Turns off faucet with paper towel.			
14. Applies non-petroleum–based hand lotion or skin protectant.			
Using Alcohol-Based Handrub			
1. If hands are soiled, washes them with soap and water.			
2. Applies a sufficient quantity of antiseptic solution to cover the hands and wrists.			
3. Rubs solution on all surfaces of fingers and hands.			
4. Continues rubbing until hands are dry.			

Recommendation: Pass _____ Needs more practice _____

Student: _____   Date: _____

Instructor: _____   Date: _____

PROCEDURE CHECKLIST
Chapter 20: Preparing and Maintaining a Sterile Field

Check (✓) Yes or No

PROCEDURE STEPS	Yes	No	COMMENTS
Preparing a Sterile Field With Commercial Package			
1. Places sterile package on a clean, dry surface.			

2. Opens flaps in this order to create a sterile field:
    a. Opens the flap farthest from own body.
    b. Opens side flaps.
    c. Opens flap nearest body.			

3. Treats as unsterile the area 1 inch from all edges of the wrapper, and any area hanging over the edge of the table.			
Preparing a Sterile Field with Fabric or Paper-Wrapped Package			
4. Checks and removes chemical indicator strip.			
5. Removes outer wrapper and places inner package on a clean, dry surface.			
6. Opens inner wrapper following the same technique described in #2 above.			
Preparing a Sterile Drape			
7. Places package on a clean, dry surface.			
8. Holds the edge of the package flap down toward the table and grasps the top edge of the package and peels back.			
9. Picks up sterile drape by the corner and allows it to fall open without touching unsterile surfaces.			
10. Places drape on a clean, dry surface, touching only the edge of the drape.			
11. Does not fan the drape.			
Adding Supplies to a Sterile Field			
12. Using the nondominant hand, peels back the wrapper in which the item is wrapped, creating a sterile barrier field with the inside of the wrapper.			
13. Holding the contents through the wrapper, several inches above the field, allows the supplies to drop onto the field inside the 1-inch border of the sterile field.			
14. Does not let arms pass over the sterile field; does not touch supplies with nonsterile hands.			
15. Disposes of wrapper and continues opening any needed supplies for the procedure.			

PROCEDURE STEPS	Yes	No	COMMENTS
Adding Sterile Solutions to a Sterile Field			
16. If sterile field is fabric or otherwise at risk for strikethrough, uses a sterile bowl or receptacle. It may be added to the field by unwrapping as described in the preceding section.			
17. Places sterile bowl near the edge of the sterile field.			
18. Checks that sterile solution is correct and not expired.			
19. Removes cap off solution bottle by lifting directly up.			
20. If cap will be reused, sets it upside down on a clean area.			
21. Holds bottle of solution 4 to 6 inches above the bowl to pour needed amount into the bowl.			
Other			
22. Does not leave a sterile field unattended or outside field of vision.			

Recommendation: Pass _____ Needs more practice _____

Student: _____   Date: _____

Instructor: _____   Date: _____

PROCEDURE CHECKLIST
Chapter 20: Removing Personal Protective Equipment (PPE)

Check (✓) Yes or No

PROCEDURE STEPS	Yes	No	COMMENTS
Removes PPE in the following order:			
1. If wearing a gown, unties waist ties.			
2. Removes one glove by grasping the cuff of the glove and pulling down so the glove turns inside out. Holds the glove removed in the remaining gloved hand.			
3. Slips fingers of ungloved hand inside the cuff of the other glove; pulls glove off inside out, turning it over to enclose the first glove. Does not touch self with contaminated surface of either glove.			
4. Holds contaminated gloves away from body.			
5. Disposes of gloves in a designated waste receptacle.			
6. Releases neck ties of gown, allowing gown to fall forward.			
7. Grasps gown inside of neck and peels down off arms so that the inside of the gown faces outward			
8. Holding gown away from body, discards. Does not contaminate clothing with dirty gown.			
9. Removes mask or face shield by untying lower ties first; unties upper ties next; disposes in designated waste receptacle.			

Recommendation: Pass _____ Needs more practice _____

Student: _____   Date: _____

Instructor: _____   Date: _____

Check (✓) Yes or No

PROCEDURE STEPS	Yes	No	COMMENTS
1. Applies surgical shoe covers, cap, and face mask before the scrub.			
2. Ensures that sterile gloves, gown, and towel are set up for use after the scrub.			
2. Follows agency policy for length of scrub and type of cleansing agent used (scrub typically takes 2 to 6 minutes).			
3. Follows agency policy regarding fingernail polish.			
4. Avoids chipped polish or artificial nails.			
Pre-wash			
5. Turns on water using knee or foot controls.			
6. Adjusts water temperature to warm.			
7. Wets hands and forearms from elbows to fingertips.			
8. Keeps hands above elbows and away from body.			
9. Applies liberal amount of soap.			
10. Lathers well to 2 inches above the elbow.			
11. Does not touch inside of sink.			
12. Removes debris from under nails, using nail file under running water.			
13. Rinses hands and arms, keeping hands above elbows.			
(Alternatively: Uses antibacterial gel, per agency policy; does not rinse gel.)			
Surgical Scrub Using Alcohol-Based Surgical Scrub Product			
14. Uses indicated amount.			
15. Rubs on all surfaces of hands, nails, and arms to 2 inches above the elbow.			
16. Allows hand-rub to dry completely before donning sterile gloves.			
Surgical Scrub Using Antimicrobial Soap			
17. Wets scrub brush and applies a generous amount of antimicrobial soap if not already in brush.			
18. Using a circular motion, scrubs all the surfaces of one hand and arm.			

PROCEDURE STEPS	Yes	No	COMMENTS
19. Scrubs at least 10 strokes on each nail, all sides of fingers, and each side of the hand. Uses at least 10 strokes each for the lower, middle, and upper areas of the forearm.			
20. Rinses brush and reapplies antimicrobial soap. Repeats scrub on the other hand and arm.			
21. Rinses hands and arms, keeping fingertips higher than elbows			
22. Grasps sterile towel and backs away from sterile field.			
23. Leans forward slightly and allows towel to fall open, being careful not to let it touch the uniform.			
24. Uses one end of towel to dry one hand and arm; uses opposite end to dry other hand and arm.			
25. Makes certain skin is thoroughly dry before donning sterile gloves.			

Recommendation: Pass _____ Needs more practice _____

Student: _____ Date: _____

Instructor: _____ Date: _____

Check (✓) Yes or No

PROCEDURE STEPS	Yes	No	COMMENTS
1. Places sensor pads in appropriate position (e.g., under patient's buttocks, on horizontal part of the leg).			
2. Connects control unit to the sensor pad.			
3. Connects control unit to the nurse call system, if possible.			
4. Disconnects or turns off alarm prior to assisting patient out of bed or chair.			
5. Reactivates alarm after assisting the patient back to bed or chair.			

Recommendation: Pass _____ Needs more practice _____

Student: _____   Date: _____

Instructor: _____   Date: _____

PROCEDURE CHECKLIST
Chapter 21: Using Restraints

Check (✓) Yes or No

PROCEDURE STEPS	Yes	No	COMMENTS
1. Follows agency policy and state laws for using restraints.			

2. Follows Medicare standards if applicable. Medicare standards allow for restraints only if the patient:
    a. is a danger to self or others.
    b. must be immobilized temporarily to perform a procedure.			

Applying Restraints			
3. Obtains properly sized restraint.			
4. Pads bony prominences before applying restraint.			
5. Ties and knots so that restraints can be released quickly in an emergency (e.g., half-bow).			
6. Does not tie restraints to a side rail; ties to bed frame or chair frame.			
7. Adjusts restraint to maintain good body alignment, comfort, and safety.			
8. Assesses that restraints are snug enough to prevent them from slipping off, but not tight enough to impair blood circulation (e.g., should be able to slide 2 fingers under a wrist or ankle restraint).			
Caring for Patient in Restraints			
9. At least every 2 hours, releases restraints and provides skin care, passive and active range of motion, ambulation, and toileting.			
10. Checks restraints every 30 minutes.			
11. At least every 2 hours, assesses circulation, skin integrity, and need for continuing restraint.			

Recommendation: Pass _____Needs more practice _____

Student: _____   Date: _____

Instructor: _____   Date: _____

Check (✓) Yes or No

PROCEDURE STEPS	Yes	No	COMMENTS
1. Uses warm, not hot, water (105°F or 41°C).			
2. Changes water before cleansing the perineum and whenever the water becomes dirty or cool.			
3. Drapes patient to provide privacy and prevent chilling.			
4. Removes soiled linens without exposing the patient.			
5. Removes patient's gown without exposing patient; exposes just the part of the body being bathed.			
6. If patient has an IV, removes the gown first from the arm without the IV; replaces gown on the affected arm first; does not disconnect the IV tubing; keeps IV container above level of patient's arm.			
7. Modifies procedure or stops temporarily if patient becomes tired.			
8. Follows principle of "head to toe."			
9. Follows principle of "clean to dirty."			
10. Washes extremities from distal to proximal.			
11. While bathing, keeps loose ends of washcloth from dragging across the skin and wrings out excess water.			
12. Supports joints when bathing.			
13. Rinses well if using soap.			
14. Pats dry to protect the skin.			
15. Dries thoroughly between the toes.			
16. Changes water and uses a clean washcloth to wash the perineal area.			
17. Dons procedure gloves to wash rectal area; removes any fecal matter with tissues prior to using washcloth.			
18. Applies deodorant, lotion, and/or powder as desired or as needed.			
19. Provides a back rub if not contraindicated.			
20. When finished, repositions patient and changes bed linen as needed.			

Recommendation: Pass _____ Needs more practice _____

Student: _____   Date: _____

Instructor: _____   Date: _____

Check (✓) Yes or No

PROCEDURE STEPS	Yes	No	COMMENTS
1. Peels open label on commercial bath without completely removing it. (Alternatively, places 8 or 10 washcloths in a plastic bag and covers with water.)			
2. Heats in microwave for no longer than 1 minute. Temperature should be approximately 105°F or 41°C.			
3. Drapes patient to provide privacy and prevent chilling.			
4. Removes soiled linens without exposing the patient.			
5. Removes patient's gown without exposing patient; exposes just the part of the body being bathed.			
6. If patient has an IV, removes the gown first from the arm without the IV; replaces gown on the affected arm first.			
7. Uses one washcloth for each body area; discards each washcloth after use (if disposable).			
7. Modifies procedure or stops temporarily if patient becomes tired.			
8. Follows principle of "head to toe."			
9. Follows principle of "clean to dirty."			
10. Washes extremities from distal to proximal.			
11. While bathing, keeps loose ends of washcloth from dragging across the skin and wrings out excess water.			
12. Supports joints when bathing.			
13. Pats dry to protect the skin.			
14. Dries thoroughly between the toes.			
15. Dons procedure gloves to wash rectal area; removes any fecal matter with tissues prior to using washcloth.			
16 Applies deodorant, lotion, and/or powder as desired or as needed.			
17. Provides a back rub if not contraindicated.			
18. When finished, repositions patient, and changes bed linen as needed.			

Recommendation: Pass _____ Needs more practice _____

Student: _____   Date: _____

Instructor: _____   Date: _____

PROCEDURE CHECKLIST
Chapter 22: Bathing: Providing a Towel Bath

Check (✓) Yes or No

PROCEDURE STEPS	Yes	No	COMMENTS
1. Places bath blanket, bath towel, and 2 or 3 washcloths in large plastic bag.			
2. Fills pitcher with approximately 2000 mL warm water, adds nonrinse soap or commercial solution to the water, and pours solution into the bag over the bath blanket, towel, and washcloths.			
3. Uses warm, not hot, water (105°F or 41°C).			
4. Places dry bath blanket over patient, pulls down bed linens, without exposing the patient.			
5. Removes patient's gown without exposing patient.			
6. If patient has an IV, removes the gown first from the arm without the IV; replaces gown on the affected arm first.			
7. Replaces dry blanket with wet blanket: a. Squeezes out excess water so it does not drip.			
b. Pushes dry blanket down to patient's waist and places wet blanket on the chest, continues to unfold wet blanket in this manner, keeping dry blanket dry.			
8. Bathes patient beginning at the feet and working toward the head.			
9. Uses wet blanket to wash legs, abdomen, and chest.			
10. As bathing is done, replaces wet blanket with the dry one.			
11. Uses one wash cloth to wash patient's face, neck, and ears.			
12. Rolls client to one side and uses wet towel to wash the back and then the buttocks.			
13. Dons procedure gloves to wash rectal area; removes any fecal matter with tissues prior to using washcloth.			
14. Using washcloths, provides perineal care.			
15. Supports joints when bathing.			
16. Pats dry with dry towel, as needed; dries thoroughly between the toes.			
17. Applies deodorant, lotion, and/or powder as desired or as needed.			

PROCEDURE STEPS	Yes	No	COMMENTS
18. Provides a back rub if not contraindicated.			
19. When finished, repositions patient, and changes bed linen as needed.			

Recommendation: Pass _____ Needs more practice _____

Student: _____   Date: _____

Instructor: _____   Date: _____

PROCEDURE CHECKLIST
Chapter 22: Brushing and Flossing the Teeth

Check (✓) Yes or No

PROCEDURE STEPS	Yes	No	COMMENTS
1. Positions patient to prevent aspiration (sitting or side-lying), as needed.			
2. Sets up suction, if needed.			
3. For self-care, arranges supplies within patient's reach and assists only as needed.			
Nurse-Administered Brushing and Flossing			
4. Places towel across patient's chest.			
5. Moistens toothbrush and applies small amount of toothpaste			
6. Places, holds, or has patient hold, the emesis basin under his chin			
7. Brushes teeth, holding bristles at a 45° angle.			
a. Uses short, circular motions.			
b. Brushes all surfaces of the teeth from gum line to crown.			
c. If patient is at risk for choking, suctions secretions as needed.			
d. Gently brushes the patient's tongue.			

8. Flosses teeth using floss holder or using the following technique:
    a. Wraps one end of the floss around the middle finger of each hand.
    b. Stretches the floss between thumbs and index fingers and moves the floss up and down against each tooth.
    c. Flosses between and around all teeth.			

9. Assists patient in rinsing mouth, suctioning as needed if patient is frail. Or asks the patient to rinse vigorously and spit the water into the emesis basin.			
10. Offers a mild or dilute mouthwash and applies lip moisturizer if desired.			
11. Repositions patient as needed.			

Recommendation: Pass _____ Needs more practice _____

Student: _____   Date: _____

Instructor: _____   Date: _____

PROCEDURE CHECKLIST
Chapter 22: Making an Occupied Bed

Check (✓) Yes or No

PROCEDURE STEPS	Yes	No	COMMENTS
NOTE: This checklist is designed to evaluate making an occupied bed separately from giving a bed bath. If linen change is done at the same time as the bed bath, some of these steps will vary.			
1. Positions bed flat if possible, and raises to appropriate working height. Lowers the side rail nearest the nurse.			
2. Loosens all the bedding. Disconnects call device and removes the patient's personal items from the bed.			
3. Checks that no tubes are entangled in the bed linens.			
4. Removes blanket and/or bedspread; if clean, folds and places on a clean area. Does not place clean linen on another patient's bed or furniture.			
5a. Slides patient to far side of the bed, places in side-lying position facing the side rail.			
5b. Places pillow under patients head; if needed, places a pillow between patient and side rail.			
6a. Rolls or tightly fan-folds the soiled linens toward patient's back; tucks the roll slightly under the patient.			
6b. Covers any moist areas of the soiled linen with a waterproof pad.			
7a. Places clean bottom sheet and drawsheet on near side of the mattress, with the center vertical fold at the center of the bed.			
7b. Fanfolds the half of the clean linen that is to be used on the far side, folding it as close to the patient as possible and tucking it under the dirty linen.			
7c. Tucks the lower edges of clean linen under the mattress. Smoothes out all wrinkles.			
8a. Explains to patient that he will be rolling over a "lump."			
8b. Rolls patient over dirty linen and gently pulls patient toward her so the patient rolls onto the clean linen.			
9. Raises side rail on "clean" side of the bed.			

PROCEDURE STEPS	Yes	No	COMMENTS
9a. Moves pillows to the clean side of the bed; positions patient side-lying near the bed rail on the clean side.			
10. Moves to opposite side of bed; lowers bedrail.			
11. Pulls soiled linen from away from patient. Removes from bed and places in laundry bag or hamper without contaminating uniform.			
12. Does not put soiled linen on the floor or other surfaces.			
13. Pulls clean linens through to the unmade side of the bed, and tucks them in.			
14. Pulls linens taut, starting with the middle section.			
15. Assists patient to a supine position close to the center of the mattress.			
16. Places top sheet and bedspread along one side of the mattress; tucks them in at the same time, then moves to opposite side of the bed.			
17. After making both sides of the bed, at the head of the bed, folds sheet down over bedspread.			
18. At foot of the bed, makes a small pleat in the top sheet and bedspread; then tucks in bottom of sheet and bedspread at the same time.			
19. Miters corners neatly.			
20. Changes pillowcases: grasps middle of closed end of pillowcase; reaches through pillowcase and grasps end of pillow; pulls pillow back through pillowcase. Does not hold pillow under arm or chin.			
21. Returns bed to low position, raises side rails, and attaches call light within patient's reach.			
22. Positions bedside table and over-bed table within patient's reach.			

Recommendation: Pass _____ Needs more practice _____

Student: _____   Date: _____

Instructor: _____   Date: _____

PROCEDURE CHECKLIST
Chapter 22: Making an Unoccupied Bed

Check (✓) Yes or No

PROCEDURE STEPS	Yes	No	COMMENTS
1. Assists patient to chair; provides robe/blanket if needed.			
2. Positions bed flat, raises to working height, lowers side rails.			
3. Folds and places clean bedspread and/or blanket on clean area. Does not place clean linen on another patient's bed or furniture.			
4. Removes all sheets and pillowcases; places in laundry bag or hamper without contaminating uniform.			
5. Does not place linen on the floor.			
6. Removes and replaces linens on one side of the bed at a time, to save steps.			
7. Does not "shake" or "fan" linens.			
8. For flat bottom sheet, allows at least 10 inches to hang over at top and sides for tuck-in.			
9. Smoothes wrinkles from bottom sheet.			
10. If there is a draw sheet, tucks it and draws it tight.			
11. Replaces waterproof pad if one is being used.			
12. Places top sheet and bedspread along one side of the mattress; tucks them in at the same time, using a mitered corner. Then moves to opposite side of the bed.			
13. After making both sides of the bed, at the head of the bed, folds sheet down over bedspread.			
14. At foot of the bed, makes a small pleat in the top sheet and bedspread.			
15. Fanfolds top sheet and bedspread back to the foot of the bed.			
16. Changes pillowcases: grasps middle of closed end of pillowcase; reaches through pillowcase and grasps end of pillow; pulls pillow back through pillowcase. Does not hold pillow under arm or chin.			
17. Assists client back to bed.			
18. Places call signal within reach.			
19. Places bedside table and over-bed table so they are accessible to the client.			

Recommendation: Pass _____ Needs more practice_____

Student: _____   Date: _____

Instructor: _____   Date: _____

PROCEDURE CHECKLIST
Chapter 22: Providing Beard and Mustache Care

Check (✓) Yes or No

PROCEDURE STEPS	Yes	No	COMMENTS
1. Trims beard and mustache when dry.			
2. Trims conservatively; cutting too little rather than too much.			
3. If using comb and scissors, cuts the hair on the outside of the comb.			
4. If using beard trimmer, adjusts the guide to the correct length.			
5. Trims beard from in front of the ear to the chin on one side, then repeats on the other.			
6. Mustache: Combs straight down, then starts in the middle and trims first toward one side of the mouth, then the other. Does not trim top of mustache.			
7. Defines beard line with the scissors or a beard trimmer; or shaves the neck to define the beard line.			
8. Shampoos facial hair as needed; rinses well; dries with towel. Applies conditioner if patient desires.			
9. Combs the beard and mustache with a wide-toothed comb or brush.			

Recommendation: Pass _____ Needs more practice _____

Student: _____   Date: _____

Instructor: _____   Date: _____

PROCEDURE CHECKLIST
Chapter 22: Providing Denture Care

Check (✓) Yes or No

PROCEDURE STEPS	Yes	No	COMMENTS
1. Removes upper denture before lower denture.			
2. To remove upper denture, with a gauze pad, grasps denture with thumb and forefinger and moves gently up and down. Tilts denture slightly to one side to remove it without stretching the lips.			
3. To remove lower denture, uses thumbs to gently push up on denture at gum line to release from lower jaw. Grasps denture with thumb and forefinger and tilts to remove from patient's mouth.			
4. Places each denture in denture cup after removing.			
5. Places towel or basin of water in sink to prevent damage to dentures.			
6. Cleanses dentures under cool running water.			
7. Applies small amount of toothpaste to stiff-bristled toothbrush; brushes all surfaces of each denture; rinses thoroughly with cool water. **Alternatively**, soaks stained dentures in a commercial cleaner, following manufacturer's instructions.			
8. Inspects dentures for rough, worn, or sharp edges before replacing.			
9. Inspects the mouth under the dentures for redness, irritation, lesions, or infection before replacing dentures.			
10. Applies denture adhesive as needed or as desired by patient.			
11. Replaces upper denture before lower denture.			
12. Moistens upper denture, if dry; inserts at a slight tilt, and presses it up against the roof of the mouth.			
13. Moistens bottom denture, if dry; inserts denture, rotating as it is placed in the patient's mouth.			
14. If patient does not wish to wear the dentures, covers them with water in a denture container with a lid. Labels the container with patient's name and agency identifying number.			
15. Offers mouthwash.			

Recommendation: Pass _____ Needs more practice _____

Student: _____   Date: _____

Instructor: _____   Date: _____

PROCEDURE CHECKLIST
Chapter 22: Providing Foot Care

Check (✓) Yes or No

PROCEDURE STEPS	Yes	No	COMMENTS
1. Has patient sit in a chair or places in semi-Fowler's position with a pillow under the knees.			
2. Fills basin half-full with warm water (approximately 105° to 110°F or 40° to 43°C).			
3. Changes water if it becomes cool or dirty.			
4. Inspects feet thoroughly for skin integrity, circulation, and edema; checks between toes.			
5. Places waterproof pad or bath towel under the feet and basin.			
6. Soaks each foot, one at a time, for 5 to 20 minutes (contraindicated for patients with diabetes of peripheral vascular disease).			
7. Changes water between feet, if necessary.			
8. Cleans feet with mild soap; cleans toenails with orange stick while foot is still in the water; pushes cuticles back with orange stick.			
9. Rinses (or uses rinse-free soap) and dries well (especially between toes).			
10. Trims nails straight across with toenail clippers, unless contraindicated by patient's condition or by institutional policy.			
11. Files nails with emery board.			
12. Lightly applies cream, lotion, or foot powder. Does not apply cream or lotion between the toes.			
13. Ensures that footwear and bedding are not irritating to feet; applies protective devices such as lamb's wool, if needed. Uses bed cradle to keep linens off the feet if patient has an injury, lesions, pain, or is at high risk for impaired skin integrity.			

Recommendation: Pass _____ Needs more practice _____

Student: _____   Date: _____

Instructor: _____   Date: _____

PROCEDURE CHECKLIST
Chapter 22: Providing Oral Care for an Unconscious Patient

Check (✓) Yes or No

PROCEDURE STEPS	Yes	No	COMMENTS
1. Determines whether the patient has dentures or partial plate; assesses gag reflex.			
2. Positions side-lying, head turned to side and, if possible, with head of bed lowered slightly.			
3. Sets up suction: attaches tubing and tonsil-tip suction, checks suction.			
4. Brushes patient's teeth.			
a. Places waterproof pad and then towel under patient's cheek and chin.			
b. Places emesis basin under patient's cheek.			
c. Moistens toothbrush and applies a small amount of toothpaste.			
d. Uses padded tongue blade or bite-block to hold mouth open.			
e. Brushes teeth, holding bristles at a 45° angle to the gum line.			
f. Uses short, circular motions.			
g. Gently brushes the inner and outer surfaces of the teeth, including the gum line.			
h. Brushes the biting surface of the back teeth by holding the toothbrush perpendicular to the teeth and brushing back and forth.			
i. Brushes the patient's tongue.			
5. Draws about 10 mL of water or mouthwash (e.g., dilute hydrogen peroxide) into a syringe; ejects it gently into the side of the mouth. Allows the fluid to drain out into the basin; or suctions as needed.			
6. Cleans the tissues in the oral cavity according to agency policy.			
a. Uses foam swabs or a moistened gauze square wrapped around a tongue blade.			
b. Uses a clean swab for each area of the mouth: cheeks, tongue, roof of the mouth, and so forth.			
7. Removes basin, dries face and mouth, applies water-soluble lip moisturizer.			

PROCEDURE STEPS	Yes	No	COMMENTS

Recommendation: Pass _____ Needs more practice _____

Student: _____   Date: _____

Instructor: _____   Date: _____

PROCEDURE CHECKLIST
Chapter 22: Providing Perineal Care

Check (✓) Yes or No

PROCEDURE STEPS	Yes	No	COMMENTS
1. Assists with elimination as needed.			
2. Fills the basin or perineal wash bottle with warm water (temperature should be approximately 105°F or 41°C).			
3. Positions patient supine.			
4. Places waterproof pads under patient.			
5. If perineum is grossly soiled, places patient on a bedpan or portable sitz tub.			
6. Removes any fecal material with toilet paper.			
7. Moistens washcloth with water in the basin or sprays perineum with the perineal wash bottle.			
8. For females:			
a. Washes perineum from front to back.			
b. Uses a clean portion of the washcloth for each stroke.			
c. Cleanses the labial folds and around the urinary catheter if one is in place.			
9. For males:			
a. Retracts the foreskin, if present.			
b. Cleanses the head of the penis using a circular motion.			
c. Replaces foreskin and finishes washing the shaft of the penis, using firm strokes.			
d. Washes scrotum, using a clean portion of the cloth with each stroke.			
e. Handles the scrotum gently to avoid discomfort.			
10. Cleanses skin folds thoroughly, rinses, and pats dry.			
11. If perineal care is not being done as part of the bath, also cleans the anal area by having patient turn to the side and washing, rinsing, and drying the area as needed.			
12. Applies skin protectants as needed. Uses powder only if patient requests it.			
13. If patient has an indwelling catheter, provides special catheter care as prescribed by agency policy. Dons clean gloves before special catheter care.			

PROCEDURE STEPS	Yes	No	COMMENTS
14. Repositions and covers patient.			
15. Removes and appropriately discards soiled gloves.			

Recommendation: Pass _____ Needs more practice _____

Student: _____   Date: _____

Instructor: _____   Date: _____

Check (✓) Yes or No

PROCEDURE STEPS	Yes	No	COMMENTS
1. Instills 1–2 drops of wetting solution.			
2. Removes lenses gently, using finger pads, not fingernails.			
3. Cleanses, rinses, and places the first-removed lens in its designated cup before removing the second lens.			
4. Cleans and stores lenses in sterile solution; uses saline if lens solution is not available.			
5. Cleans lenses according to instructions on the cleansing solution bottle.			
6. Rinses after cleansing, with contact lens solution or sterile saline.			
7. Places lenses in lens case with soaking solution or sterile saline.			
8. Uses marked container to store lenses, or marks the container "L" and "R" to identify the correct eye.			
Removing Hard or Gas Permeable Lenses			
9a. If the lens is not centered over the cornea, places finger on the lower eyelid and applies gentle pressure to move it into position.			
9b. Places index finger at the outer corner of the eye and gently pulls sideways toward the ear; positions other hand below the eye to "catch" the lens.			
9c. Asks the patient to blink. As the skin tightens, the contact will "pop" out.			
Alternatively:			
9d. Gently pulls top eyelid up and lower lid down so they are beyond the top and bottom edges of the lens.			
9e. Then gently presses the lower eyelid up against the bottom of the lens; when lens is slightly tipped, moves the eyelids together.			

PROCEDURE STEPS	Yes	No	COMMENTS
Removing Soft Contact Lenses			
10a. Holds the eye open with the nondominant hand.			
10b. Gently places tip of index finger on the lens and slides it down off the pupil into the white area of the eye.			
10c. Using thumb and index fingerpads (gloved), gently pinches the lens and lifts it straight up off the eye.			

Recommendation: Pass _____ Needs more practice _____

Student: _____   Date: _____

Instructor: _____   Date: _____

Check (✓) Yes or No

PROCEDURE STEPS	Yes	No	COMMENTS
1. With input from patient, as able, identifies hair care products needed for the procedure.			
2. Unless contraindicated, lowers head of the bed; removes pillow from under patient's neck, and places it under her shoulders.			
3. Places waterproof pad or plastic trash bag under patient's shoulders and covers with towels.			
4. Places shampoo tray under patient's shoulders (or head, depending on how it is made). If using a hard plastic tray, liberally pads with towels. An inflatable shampoo tray needs minimal padding. Ensures that the tray will drain into the washbasin or other receptacle.			
5. Folds the top linens down to the patient's waist and covers her upper body with a bath blanket.			
6. If lesions or infestation are present, dons procedure gloves at this step.			
7. Works fingers through hair or combs hair to remove tangles prior to washing.			
8. Washes the hair. a. Wets the hair using warm water then applies shampoo and lathers well.			
b. Works from the scalp out and from the front to the back of the head.			
c. Gently lifts the patient's head to rub the back of the head.			
9. Rinses thoroughly.			
10. If desired, applies conditioner to the hair. Conditioner should be used for patients with hair that tangles easily, such as dry, long, curly, or kinky hair. Rinses if needed.			
11. Removes the tray and blots dry hair with towel. Does not use circular motions to dry the hair.			
12. Combs or brushes hair to remove tangles, starting at the ends and working toward the scalp.			
13. If desired, dries hair with hair dryer at a medium temperature.			
Variation: Shampooing the Hair of African-American Clients			
14. Dons procedure gloves if lesions or infestations are present.			

PROCEDURE STEPS	Yes	No	COMMENTS
15. If the hair is in cornrows or braids, does not take out the braids to wash the hair.			
16. Handles the patient's hair very gently, being careful not to pull on the hair.			
17. When shampooing, threads fingers through the hair from the scalp out to the ends. Does not massage the hair in circular motions.			
18. Uses a conditioner on the hair.			
19. Does not use a brush or fine-toothed comb on patient's hair. Uses a wide-toothed comb or hair pick.			

a. Parts the hair into four sections and, using a wide-toothed comb or hair pick, begins combing near the ends of the hair, working through each section.
     b. Uses additional moisturizer to help soften and ease combing.
     c. Does not pull on the hair.
     d. Lets hair air-dry, if possible.			

Variation: Shampooing the Hair Using Rinse-Free Shampoo			
20. If possible, elevates the head of the bed.			
21. Places bath towel under patient's shoulders.			
22. Dons procedure gloves if lesions or infestations are present.			
23. Works fingers through hair or combs hair to remove tangles prior to washing. If the patient has her hair in small braids, does not take out the braids to wash the hair. Black curly hair is fragile, so handles it gently.			
24. Applies rinse-free shampoo to thoroughly wet the hair.			
25. Works through hair, from scalp down to ends.			
26. Dries with bath towel.			
Variation: Shampooing the Hair Using Rinse-Free Shampoo Cap			
27. Warms the shampoo cap using a water bath or microwave, according to package instructions.			
28. Checks temperature before placing on patient's head.			
29. Places cap on patient's hair and massages gently.			
30. Removes cap and towel dries the patient's hair.			

Recommendation: Pass _____ Needs more practice _____

Student: _____ Date: _____

Instructor: _____ Date: _____

PROCEDURE CHECKLIST
Chapter 22: Shaving a Patient

Check (✓) Yes or No

PROCEDURE STEPS	Yes	No	COMMENTS
1. Uses patient's chosen shaving method (e.g., safety or electric razor).			
2. Places warm, damp face towel on face for 1 to 2 minutes.			
3. Applies shaving cream with fingers or shaving brush; lathers well for 1 to 2 minutes.			
4a. Pulls skin taut with nondominant hand.			
4b. If using safety razor, holds blade at 45° angle.			
4c. Gently pulls razor across skin.			
4d. Shaves face and neck in the same direction as hair growth.			
4e. Uses short strokes.			
4f. Begins at sideburns and works down to chin on each side; then shaves the neck; last, shaves chin and upper lip.			
5. Rinses razor frequently while shaving.			
6. When finished, rinses face with cool water and gently pats dry.			
7. Applies after-shave lotion if patient desires.			

Recommendation: Pass _____ Needs more practice _____

Student: _____   Date: _____

Instructor: _____   Date: _____

Chapter 23: Medication Guidelines
Steps to Follow for All Medications, Regardless of Type or Route

Check (✓) Yes or No

PROCEDURE STEPS	Yes	No	COMMENTS
1. *First Check*: Checks medication order on MAR against physician's order (patient name, identification number, medication, dose, route, time, and allergies).			
2. Follows agency policies for medication administration, including the time frame for medication administration. Most agencies allow medications to be given 30 minutes before or 30 minutes after the time indicated in the MAR.			
3. Knows drug information, including drug action, purpose, recommended dosage, time of onset and peak action, common side effects, contraindications, drug interactions, and nursing implications.			
4. Determines if medication dosage is appropriate for patient's age and weight.			
5. Identifies any special considerations for medication preparation and administration, such as can the medication be crushed or a capsule opened, or should medication be administered with food or on an empty stomach.			
6. Checks expiration date of medication.			
7. *Second Check*: When preparing medication, verifies correct medication, dose, time, route, and expiration date.			
8. Calculates dosage accurately.			
9. Locks medication cart after removing medication.			
10. *Third Check*: At the bedside, verifies correct patient (using two methods of identification, including armband), medication, expiration date, dose, route, time, and presence of drug allergies.			
11. Remains with the patient until sure he has taken the medication.			
12. Does not leave medication unattended at bedside.			
13. Reassesses for therapeutic and side effects.			
14. Teaches patient about the medication as needed.			

Recommendation: Pass _____ Needs more practice _____

Student: _____   Date: _____

Instructor: _____   Date: _____

PROCEDURE CHECKLIST
Chapter 23: Adding Medications to Intravenous Fluids

Check (✓) Yes or No

PROCEDURE STEPS	Yes	No	COMMENTS
1. Prepares and administers medications according to "Medication Guidelines: Steps to Follow for All Medications."			
2. Determines whether the ordered medication(s) are compatible with the intravenous solution and with each other.			
3. Recaps needles throughout, using a needle-capping device or approved one-handed technique that has a low risk of contaminating the sterile needle (see Procedure Checklist Chapter 23: Recapping Needles Using One-Handed Technique).			
4. Correctly calculates the amount of medication to be instilled into the intravenous solution.			
5a. Removes any protective covers and inspects the bag/bottle for leaks, tears, or cracks.			
5b. Inspects the fluid for clarity, color, and presence of any particulate matter.			
5c. Checks the expiration date.			
6. Using the appropriate technique, draws up the ordered medication (see Procedure Checklist Chapter 23: Preparing and Drawing Up Medications from Ampules; Procedure Checklist Chapter 23: Preparing and Drawing Up Medications from Vials; Procedure Checklist Chapter 23: Missing Medications in One Syringe, Using Two Vials; Procedure Checklist Chapter 23: Mixing Medications in One Syringe, Using One Ampule and Vial; and Procedure Checklist Chapter 23: Mixing Medications in One Syringe, Using a Prefilled Cartridge and Single-Dose Vial—For Intravenous Administration).			
Adding Medication to a New IV Bag or Bottle			
7. Cleanses the injection port on the bag with an antimicrobial swab.			
8. Removes the cap from the syringe, inserts needle or the needleless vial access device into the injection port and injects the medication into the bag, maintaining aseptic technique.			
9. Removes syringe from injection port; if using a needle, disposes of syringe and needle.			
10. Mixes the intravenous solution and medication by gently turning the bag from end to end.			

PROCEDURE STEPS	Yes	No	COMMENTS
11. Places label on bag so that it can be read when the bag is hung.			
12. Makes sure the label does not cover the solution label or volume marks.			
13. Disposes of used equipment, syringe, or needleless access device, appropriately.			
Adding Medication to an Infusing IV			
14. Follows Steps 1–6, preceding.			
15. Determines compatibility of medication and existing solution.			
16. Notes volume remaining in existing IV and amount needed for dilution of medication (solution must be adequate to dilute the medication).			
17. Clamps the running IV line.			
18. Cleanses IV additive port with antimicrobial swab.			
19. Removes cap from syringe; inserts needle or needleless vial access device into the injection port; injects medication in to the IV bag; maintains aseptic technique. If using a needle, withdraws needle from injection port and disposes of needle and syringe safely.			
20. Mixes IV solution and medication by gently turning the bag from end to end. Keeps the bag above the level of the patient's IV insertion site.			
21. Places label on bag so that it can be read when the bag is hung.			
22. Makes sure the label does not cover the solution label or volume marks.			
23. Unclamps IV line and runs IV at prescribed rate.			
24. Disposes of used equipment, syringe, or needleless access device, appropriately.			

Recommendation: Pass _____ Needs more practice _____

Student: _____   Date: _____

Instructor: _____   Date: _____

Check (✓) Yes or No

PROCEDURE STEPS	Yes	No	COMMENTS
1. Prepares and administers medications according to "Medication Guidelines: Steps to Follow for All Medications."			
2. Selects and correctly locates site for injection. Usual sites are the ventral surface of the forearm and upper back. The upper chest may also be used.			
3. Assists patient to comfortable position. If using forearm, has patient extend and supinate arm on a flat surface. If using upper back, has patient lie prone or lean forward over a table or the back of a chair.			
4. Cleanses injection site with alcohol prep pad by circling from the center of the site outward.			
5. Allows site to dry before administering the injection.			
6. Dons procedure gloves.			
7. Holds syringe between thumb and index finger of dominant hand parallel to skin; removes needle cap.			

8. With the nondominant hand, holds skin taut by one of the following methods:
    a. If using forearm, may be able to place hand under the arm and pull the skin tight with thumb and fingers.
    b. Stretching skin between thumb and index finger.
    c. Pulling the skin toward the wrist or down with one finger.			

9. While holding the skin taut with the nondominant hand, holds syringe in dominant hand with the bevel up and parallel to the patient's skin at a 5° to 15° angle.			
10. Inserts the needle slowly and advances approximately 1/8 inch (3 mm) so that the entire bevel is covered. Bevel should be visible just under the skin.			
11. Releases the taut skin and holds syringe stable with nondominant hand. Does not aspirate.			
12. Slowly injects the solution. A pale wheal, about 6–10 mm (1/4 inch) in diameter should appear over the needle bevel.			
13. Removes needle, engages safety needle device, and disposes in biohazard puncture-proof container. If there is no safety device, places uncapped syringe and needle directly in biohazard puncture-proof container.			

PROCEDURE STEPS	Yes	No	COMMENTS
14. Gently blots any blood with a dry gauze pad. Does not rub or cover with an adhesive bandage.			
15. With pen, draws a 1-inch circle around the bleb/wheal.			

Recommendation: Pass _____ Needs more practice _____

Student: _____ Date: _____

Instructor: _____ Date: _____

Check (✓) Yes or No

PROCEDURE STEPS	Yes	No	COMMENTS
1. Prepares and administers medications according to "Medication Guidelines: Steps to Follow for All Medications."			

2. Selects appropriate syringe and needle, considering volume and type of medication, and patient's muscle mass.
 	
    a. Usual syringe size is 1–3 mL.
    b. Usual needle is 19–23 gauge, 1.5 inch in length.			

3. Selects a preferred site for injection and locates site correctly.			
4. If patient has received other injections, rotates sites.			

5. Positions patient so the injection site is accessible and the patient is able to relax the appropriate muscles.
 	
    a. Deltoid site: Positions patient with arm relaxed at side or resting on firm surface and completely expose upper arm.
    b. Ventrogluteal site: Position patient on side with upper hip and knee slightly flexed.
    c. Vastus lateralis: Position patient supine or sitting.
    d. Rectus femoris (because this site often causes more discomfort than others, use only if all other sites inaccessible and no other route feasible): Positions patient supine.
    e. Dorsogluteal (because the sciatic nerve and major blood vessels are located near this site, use only if all other sites, including the rectus femoris, are inaccessible and no other route feasible): Positions patient prone with toes pointing inward. Does not attempt to locate this site with the patient side-lying or standing.			

6. Cleanses injection site with alcohol prep pad (or other antiseptic swab) by circling from the center of the site outward. Places alcohol wipe on patient's skin outside the injection site, with a corner pointing to the site.			
7. Allows the site to dry before administering the injection.			
8. Dons procedure gloves.			

PROCEDURE STEPS	Yes	No	COMMENTS
9. Removes the needle cap.			
Traditional Intramuscular Method			
10. With nondominant hand, holds the skin taut by spreading the skin between the thumb and index finger.			
11. Holding the syringe between thumb and fingers of the dominant hand like a pencil or dart, inserts the needle at a 90° angle to the skin surface.			
12. Inserts needle fully.			
13. Stabilizes syringe and aspirates by pulling back on the plunger and waiting for 5 to 10 seconds. If there is a blood return, removes the needle, discards, and prepares the medication again.			
14. Still stabilizing syringe, uses thumb or index finger of dominant hand, presses plunger slowly to inject the medication (5 to 10 seconds per mL).			
15. Removes the needle smoothly along the line of insertion.			
16. Engages safety needle device, and disposes in biohazard container. If there is no safety device, places uncapped syringe and needle directly in biohazard puncture-proof container.			
17. Gently massages site with a gauze pad and applies Band-Aid as needed.			
Z-Track Administration			
18. Follows Steps 1 through 9, above.			
19. With the side of the nondominant hand displaces the skin away from the injection site, about 2.5 to 3.5cm (1 to 1.5 inches).			
20. Holding the syringe between thumb and fingers of the dominant hand like a pencil or dart, inserts the needle at a 90° angle to the skin surface.			
21. Stabilizes the syringe with thumb and forefinger of nondominant hand. Does not release the skin to stabilize the syringe.			
22. Aspirates by pulling back slightly on the plunger for 5 to 10 seconds. If a blood return is obtained, removes the needle, discards, and prepares the medication again.			

PROCEDURE STEPS	Yes	No	COMMENTS
23. Using thumb or index finger of dominant hand, presses plunger slowly to inject the medication (5 to 10 seconds per mL).			
24. Waits for 10 seconds, then removes the needle smoothly along the line of insertion; then immediately releases the skin.			
25. Engages safety needle device, and disposes in biohazard container. If there is no safety device, places uncapped syringe and needle directly in biohazard puncture-proof container.			
26. Does not massage the injection site.			

Recommendation: Pass _____ Needs more practice _____

Student: _____   Date: _____

Instructor: _____   Date: _____

Check (✓) Yes or No

PROCEDURE STEPS	Yes	No	COMMENTS
1. Prepares and administers medications according to "Medication Guidelines: Steps to Follow for All Medications."			
2. Checks compatibility of the medication with the existing intravenous solution, if one is infusing.			
3. Recaps needles throughout, using a needle capping device or approved one-handed technique that has a low risk of contaminating the sterile needle (see Procedure Checklist Chapter 29: Recapping Needles Using One-Handed Technique).			
4. Determines rate of administration for the medication.			
5. Dilutes medication if needed.			
6. Prepares medication from vial or ampule (see Procedure Checklist Chapter 23: Preparing and Drawing Up Medications from Ampules; Procedure Checklist Chapter 23: Preparing and Drawing Up Medications from Vials; Procedure Checklist Chapter 23: Mixing Medications in One Syringe, Using Two Vials; Procedure Checklist Chapter 23: Mixing Medications in One Syringe, Using One Ampule and Vial; Procedure Checklist Chapter 23: Mixing Medications in One Syringe, Using a Prefilled Cartridge and Single-Dose Vial—For Intravenous Administration).			
7. Thoroughly cleanses the injection port closest to the patient with alcohol prep pad or povidone-iodine.			
8. Inserts the medication syringe cannula into the injection port. If needleless system not available, insert syringe needle into the port.			
9. Pinches or clamps the IV tubing between the IV bag and the port.			
10. Gently aspirates by pulling back on the plunger to check for a blood return.			

PROCEDURE STEPS	Yes	No	COMMENTS
11. If blood is not returned, further assess patency of IV line by one of the following methods: a. By administering a small amount of the IV solution and monitoring for ease of administration, swelling at the IV site, or patient complaint of discomfort at the site. b. By lowering the IV bag below the level of the IV site and observing for a blood return. Does not give the IV push medication until patency of the IV site is verified.			
12. If blood is returned (or patency otherwise verified), administers a small increment of the medication while observing for reactions to the medication.			
13. Administers another increment of the medication (may pinch the tubing while injecting medication and release it when not injecting; this is optional).			
14. Repeats steps 12 and 13 until the medication has been administered over the correct amount of time.			
15. Disposes of used equipment properly.			

Recommendation: Pass _____ Needs more practice _____

Student: _____   Date: _____

Instructor: _____   Date: _____

Chapter 23: Administering IV Push Medications Through an Intermittent Device with IV Extension Tubing

Check (✓) Yes or No

PROCEDURE STEPS	Yes	No	COMMENTS
1. Prepares and administers medications according to "Medication Guidelines: Steps to Follow for All Medications."			
2. Checks compatibility of the medication with the existing intravenous solution, if one is infusing.			
3. Determines rate of administration for the medication.			
4. Dilutes medication if needed.			
5. Prepares medication from vial or ampule (see Procedure Checklist Chapter 23: Preparing and Drawing Up Medications from Ampules; Procedure Checklist Chapter 23: Preparing and Drawing Up Medications from Vials; Procedure Checklist Chapter 23: Mixing Medications in One Syringe, Using Two Vials; Procedure Checklist Chapter 23: Mixing Medications in One Syringe, Using One Ampule and Vial; and Procedure Checklist Chapter 23: Mixing Medications in One Syringe, Using a Prefilled Cartridge and Single-Dose Vial—For Intravenous Administration).			
6. Determines the amount of volume of any extension tubing attached to the access port.			
7. Dons procedure gloves and cleanses the injection port with an alcohol prep pad or povidone-iodine.			
8. Attaches flush syringe (insertion device, needle)			
9. Gently aspirates by pulling back on the plunger to check for a blood return.			
10. Does not administer medication unless patency of IV line can be established. If blood is not returned, assesses patency by administering a small amount of the flush solution and monitoring for ease of administration, swelling at the IV site, or patient complaint of discomfort at the site.			
11. If blood is returned, administers flush solution using a forward pushing motion on the syringe with a push-stop-push technique.			

PROCEDURE STEPS	Yes	No	COMMENTS
12. Continuing to hold the injection port, removes flush syringe, cleanses port with alcohol prep pad or povidone-iodine and attaches medication syringe. If using only one flush syringe, recaps needle, keeping it sterile.			
13. Administers a volume of medication equal to the volume of the extension set, and at the same rate as the flush solution was given.			
14. Administers the remainder of the medication in small increments (push-stop-push) over the correct time interval for the specific medication.			
15. Continuing to hold the injection port, removes medication syringe, cleanses port with alcohol prep pad or povidone-iodine and attaches flush syringe.			
16. Continues to administer flush solution at the same rate as the medication (Step 14) for the volume of the extension set, and then administers the remainder of the flush solution at the "flush" rate. (For example, if the extension tubing has a volume of 1.3 mL, gives the first 1.3 mL of the flush solution at the same rate as the medication.)			
17. Uses positive pressure technique when removing syringe. Continues to administer flush solution while withdrawing the syringe cannula from the injection port. Follow equipment guidelines, because some injection ports maintain positive pressure by removing the syringe and then closing the clamp. Others instruct the nurse to clamp the tubing and then remove the syringe.			
18. Properly disposes of used equipment.			

Recommendation: Pass _____ Needs more practice _____

Student: _____   Date: _____

Instructor: _____   Date: _____

PROCEDURE CHECKLIST
Chapter 23: Administering IV Push Medications Through an Intermittent Device (IV Lock) When No Extension Tubing is Attached to the Venous Access Device

Check (✓) Yes or No

PROCEDURE STEPS	Yes	No	COMMENTS
1. Prepares and administers medications according to "Medication Guidelines: Steps to Follow for All Medications."			
2. Checks compatibility of the medication with the existing intravenous solution, if one is infusing.			
3. Determines rate of administration for the medication.			
4. Dilutes medication if needed.			
5. Selects appropriate size syringe for flush solution.			
6. Prepares medication and saline (if necessary) from vial or ampule (see Procedure Checklist Chapter 23: Preparing and Drawing Up Medications from Ampules; Procedure Checklist Chapter 23: Preparing and Drawing Up Medications from Vials; Procedure Checklist Chapter 23: Missing Medications in One Syringe, Using Two Vials; Procedure Checklist Chapter 23: Mixing Medications in One Syringe, Using One Ampule and Vial; and Procedure Checklist Chapter 23: Mixing Medications in One Syringe, Using a Prefilled Cartridge and Single-Dose Vial—For Intravenous Administration).			
7. Dons procedure gloves and thoroughly cleanses the IV lock with alcohol prep pad or povidone-iodine.			
8. Inserts saline flush syringe cannula into injection port.			
9. Gently aspirates by pulling back on the plunger to check for a blood return.			
10. If blood is not returned, further assesses patency of IV line by administering a small amount of flush solution and monitoring for ease of administration, swelling at the IV site, or patient complaint of discomfort at the site. a. Does not give the IV push medication until patency of the IV site is verified.			
11. If blood is returned, administers flush solution using a forward pushing motion on the syringe with a push-stop-push technique.			
12. Continuing to hold the injection port, removes and recaps flush syringe using a one-handed method, cleanses port with alcohol prep pad or povidone-iodine and attaches medication syringe.			

PROCEDURE STEPS	Yes	No	COMMENTS
13. Administers the medication in small increments over the correct time interval.			
14. Continuing to hold the injection port, removes the medication syringe, cleanses the port with alcohol prep pad or povidone-iodine and attaches the flush syringe.			
15. Again administers the flush solution.			
16. Uses positive pressure technique when removing syringe. Continues to administer flush solution while withdrawing the syringe cannula from the injection port. (Or follows equipment guidelines for this step.)			
17. Properly disposes of used equipment.			

Recommendation: Pass _____ Needs more practice _____

Student: _____   Date: _____

Instructor: _____   Date: _____

PROCEDURE CHECKLIST
Chapter 23: Administering Medications Through an Enteral Tube

Check (✓) Yes or No

PROCEDURE STEPS	Yes	No	COMMENTS
1. Prepares and administers medications according to "Medication Guidelines: Steps to Follow for All Medications."			

2. Follows steps in Procedure Checklist Chapter 23: Administering Oral Medications.
   a. If pouring from a multi-dose container, does not touch the medication.
     b. Pours correct dosage.
     c. Breaks only scored tablets or uses pill cutter.
     d. For liquid medications, shakes bottle as necessary, maintains medical asepsis, does not drip on label, wipes only outside of bottle lip if dripping occurs. Measures at eye level.			

3. Checks to be sure medication can be crushed and given via enteral tube.			
4. Crushes tablet and mixes with approximately 20 mL water (or obtains liquid medication).			
5. If several medications are to be given, mixes each one separately.			
6. Places patient in high Fowler's position if possible.			
7. Checks nasogastric tube placement by aspirating stomach contents or measuring the pH of the aspirate, if possible. Other, less accurate, methods are injecting air into the feeding tube and auscultating, or asking the patient to speak.			
8. Checks for residual volume.			
9a. Flushes tube, uses correct type and size syringe.			
9b. To flush tube, removes bulb or plunger from syringe, attaches barrel to the tube, and pours in 20–30 mL of water.			
10. Instills medication by depressing syringe plunger or using barrel of syringe as a funnel and pouring in the medication. Smaller tubes require instilling with a 30–60 mL syringe; the medication can be poured with larger tubes.			
11. Flushes medication through tube by instilling an additional 20–30 mL of water.			

PROCEDURE STEPS	Yes	No	COMMENTS
12. If giving more than one medication, gives each separately and flushes after each.			
13. Has patient maintain sitting position (if able) for at least 30 minutes after medication administration.			

Recommendation: Pass _____ Needs more practice _____

Student: _____ Date: _____

Instructor: _____ Date: _____

PROCEDURE CHECKLIST
Chapter 23: Administering Nasal Medications

Check (✓) Yes or No

PROCEDURE STEPS	Yes	No	COMMENTS
1. Prepares and administers medications according to "Medication Guidelines: Steps to Follow for All Medications."			
2. Determines head position. Considers the indication for the medication and the patient's ability to assume the position.			
3. Asks patient to blow his nose.			
4. Positions patient: a. Nose drops or spray: To get head down and forward, has patient sit and lean forward or kneel on the bed with head dependent. b. If unable to assume one of those positions, has patient tilt his head back. c. To medicate ethmoid and sphenoid sinuses, assists patient into supine position with head over edge of the bed. Supports head. Alternatively, places a towel roll behind the shoulders, allowing the head to drop back. d. To medicate frontal and maxillary sinuses, positions as in step c, but tilts the head toward the affected side.			
5. Explains to the patient that the medication may cause some burning, tingling, or unusual taste.			
6. Has patient close one nostril and exhale; then inhale through the mouth.			
7. Administers spray or drops while the patient is inhaling through the mouth.			
8. Repeats steps 6 and 7 on other nostril.			
9. Does not touch dropper to the sides of the nostril.			
10. If nose drops are used, asks the patient to stay in the same position for approximately 5 minutes (follow manufacturer's guidelines).			
11. Instructs patient not to blow his nose for several minutes.			

Recommendation: Pass _____ Needs more practice _____

Student: _____   Date: _____

Instructor: _____   Date: _____

PROCEDURE CHECKLIST
Chapter 23: Administering Ophthalmic Medications

Check (✓) Yes or No

PROCEDURE STEPS	Yes	No	COMMENTS
1. Prepares and administers medications according to "Medication Guidelines: Steps to Follow for All Medications."			
2. If possible, assists patient to high Fowler's position with head slightly tilted back.			
3. If needed, cleans edges of eyelid from inner to outer canthus.			
Instilling Eye Drops			
4a. Holding eyedropper, rests dominant hand on patient's forehead.			
4b. With nondominant hand, pulls the lower lid down to expose the conjunctival sac.			
4c. Positions eyedropper 1/2 to 3/4 inch (13 to 19 mm) above patient's eye; does not let dropper touch the eye.			
4d. Asks patient to look up; drops correct number of drops into conjunctival sac. Does not drop onto cornea.			
4e. Asks patient to gently close and move the eyes.			
5. If medication has systemic effects, presses gently against the same side of the nose to close the lacrimal ducts for 1 to 2 minutes.			
Administering Eye Ointment			
6a. Rests dominant hand, with eye ointment, on patient's forehead.			
6b. With nondominant hand, pulls the lower lid down to expose the conjunctival sac.			
6c. Asks patient to look up.			
6d. Applies a thin strip of ointment (about 1 inch; 2 to 2.5 cm) in conjunctival sac; twists wrist to break off the strip.			
6e. Does not let tube touch the eye.			
6f. Asks patient to gently close eyes for 2 to 3 minutes.			
7. Explains that vision will be blurred for a short time.			

Recommendation: Pass _____ Needs more practice _____

Student: _____ Date: _____

Instructor: _____ Date: _____

PROCEDURE CHECKLIST
Chapter 23: Administering Oral Medications

Check (✓) Yes or No

PROCEDURE STEPS	Yes	No	COMMENTS
1. Prepares and administers medications according to "Medication Guidelines: Steps to Follow for All Medications."			
Tablets and Capsules			
2. If pouring from a multi-dose container, does not touch the medication. Pours the tablet into the cap of the bottle, then into the medication cup.			
3. Pours correct number into medication cup.			
4. If necessary to give less than a whole tablet, breaks scored tablet with hands; uses a pill cutter if necessary. Does not break unscored tablet.			
5. If drug is unit-dose, does not open package; places entire package in paper (soufflé) cup.			
6. If patient has difficulty swallowing, checks to see if the pill can be crushed. If so, mixes with soft food, such as applesauce.			
7. Pours all medications scheduled at the same time into the same cup, except uses separate cup for any medications requiring pre-administration assessment (e.g., digoxin).			
8. If patient is able to hold it, places tablet or medication cup in her hand. If unable to hold it, places medication cup to her lips and tips the pill(s) into her mouth.			
9. Provides liquid to swallow the pills.			
Sublingual Medications			
10. Places, or has patient place, the tablet under the tongue and hold there until completely dissolved.			
Buccal Medications			
11. Places, or has patient place, the tablet between cheek and teeth and hold there until completely dissolved.			
Liquids			
12. Shakes the liquid, if necessary, before opening the container.			
13. Places bottle lid upside down on the counter.			
14. Holds bottle with label in palm of the hand.			
15. Pours medication, slightly twists bottle when finished to prevent dripping.			

PROCEDURE STEPS	Yes	No	COMMENTS
16. If medication drips over bottle lip when pouring, wipes with a clean tissue or paper towel—only the outside lip of the bottle.			
17. Holds medication cup at eye level to measure dosage.			
18. Positions patient in high Fowler's position if possible; or raises head of bed as much as allowed; or uses side-lying position.			

Recommendation: Pass _____ Needs more practice _____

Student: _____   Date: _____

Instructor: _____   Date: _____

PROCEDURE CHECKLIST
Chapter 23: Administering Otic Medications

Check (✓) Yes or No

PROCEDURE STEPS	Yes	No	COMMENTS
1. Prepares and administers medications according to "Medication Guidelines: Steps to Follow for All Medications."			
2. Warms solution to be instilled (e.g., in hand or in warm, not hot, water).			
3. Assists patient to side-lying position, with appropriate ear facing up.			
4. Fills dropper with the correct amount of medication.			
5. Cleans external ear with cotton tipped applicator if needed.			
6. For infants and young children, asks another caregiver to immobilize the child while administering the medication.			
7. Straightens the ear canal. a. For patients older than 3 years, pulls pinna upward and back. b. For children less than 3 years old, pulls pinna down and back.			
8. Instills correct number of drops along the side of the ear canal.			
9. Does not touch the end of the dropper to any part of the ear.			
10. Massages or presses on the tragus of the ear.			
11. Instructs patient to remain on his side for 5 to 10 min.			
12. Places cotton loosely at the opening of the auditory canal for 15 minutes.			

Recommendation: Pass _____ Needs more practice _____

Student: _____   Date: _____

Instructor: _____   Date: _____

PROCEDURE CHECKLIST
Chapter 23: Administering Subcutaneous Medications

Check (✓) Yes or No

PROCEDURE STEPS	Yes	No	COMMENTS
1. Prepares and administers medications according to "Medication Guidelines: Steps to Follow for All Medications."			
2. Does not give more than 1 mL of medication in a site.			
3. Selects appropriate syringe and needle. In addition to considering the amount of adipose tissue: a. For insulin, must use an insulin syringe. b. For volumes less than 1 ml, uses a tuberculin (TB) syringe with a 25–27 gauge, 3/8–5/8 inch needle. c. For a volume of 1 mL, a 3 ml syringe may be used with a 25–27 gauge, 3/8–5/8 inch needle.			
4. Selects and locates an appropriate site (outer aspect of the upper arms, abdomen, anterior aspects of the thighs, and the scapular area on the upper back). Site must have adequate subcutaneous tissue. For heparin, the abdomen is the only site used.			
5. Positions patient so the injection site is accessible and patient can relax the area.			
6. Cleanses injection site with alcohol prep pad by circling from the center of the site outward.			
7. Allows the site to dry before administering the injection.			
8. Dons procedure gloves.			
9. Removes the needle cap.			
10. With nondominant hand, pinches or pulls taut the skin at the injection site. a. If client is obese or "pinch" of adipose tissue is greater than 2 inches, uses a 90° angle. b. If client is average size or "pinch" is less than 1 inch, uses 45° angle. c. If the client is obese and the adipose tissue pinches 2 inches or more, uses a longer needle and spreads the skin taut instead of pinching.			

PROCEDURE STEPS	Yes	No	COMMENTS
11. Holding the syringe between thumb and index finger of the dominant hand like a pencil or dart, inserts the needle at the appropriate angle at the into the pinched-up skinfold.			
12. Stabilizes the syringe with the fingers of the nondominant hand.			
13. Using thumb or index finger of dominant hand, presses plunger slowly to inject the medication. (Alternatively, after inserting the needle, continues to hold the barrel with the dominant hand and use nondominant hand to depress the plunger.)			
14. Removes the needle smoothly along the line of insertion.			
15. Gently blots any blood with a gauze pad. Does not massage the site.			
16. Engages needle safety device or places the uncapped syringe and needle directly into a "sharps" container.			

Recommendation: Pass _____ Needs more practice _____

Student: _____   Date: _____

Instructor: _____   Date: _____

PROCEDURE CEHCKLIST
Chapter 23: Administering Vaginal Medications

Check (✓) Yes or No

PROCEDURE STEPS	Yes	No	COMMENTS
For All Vaginal Medications			
1. Prepares and administers medications according to "Medication Guidelines: Steps to Follow for All Medications."			
2. Has patient void before procedure.			
3. Positions patient in dorsal recumbent or Sims' position.			
4. Drapes patient with bath blanket so that only the perineum is exposed.			
5. Prepares medication: a. Removes wrapper from suppository and places loosely in wrapper container. b. Or fills applicator according to manufacturer's instructions.			
6. For irrigations, uses warm solution (temperature approximately 105°F).			
7. Uses only water-soluble lubricant.			
8. Inspects and cleans around vaginal orifice.			
Administering a Suppository			
9. Applies water-soluble lubricant to the rounded end of the suppository and to gloved index finger on the dominant hand.			
10. Separates labia with gloved nondominant hand.			
11. Inserts the suppository as far as possible along the posterior vaginal wall (about 3 inches, or 8 cm). If the suppository comes with an applicator, places the suppository in the end of the applicator, inserts the applicator into the vagina and presses plunger.			
12. Has patient remain in supine position for 5 to 15 minutes. May elevate her hips on a pillow.			
Applicator Insertion of Cream, Foam, or Jelly			
13. Separates labia with nondominant hand.			
14. Inserts applicator approximately 3 inches into vagina along the posterior vaginal wall.			
15. Depresses plunger, emptying medication into vagina.			

PROCEDURE STEPS	Yes	No	COMMENTS
16. Disposes of applicator or places on paper towel if reusable.			
17. Has patient remain supine for 5 to 15 minutes.			
Vaginal Irrigation			
18. Hangs irrigation solution approximately 1 to 2 feet (30 to 60 cm) above the level of the patient's vagina.			
19. Assists patient into dorsal-recumbent position.			
20. Places waterproof pad and bedpan under patient.			
21. If using a vaginal irrigation set with tubing, opens the clamp to allow the solution to completely fill the tubing.			
22. Lubricates end of irrigation nozzle.			
23. Inserts nozzle approximately 3 inches (7 to 8 cm) into the vagina, directing it toward the sacrum.			
24. Starts the flow of the irrigation solution, rotates nozzle intermittently as solution is flowing.			
25. If labia are reddened, runs some of the solution over the labia.			
26. After all irrigating solution has been used, removes nozzle and assists patient to a sitting position on the bedpan (to drain all the solution).			
27. Removes bedpan.			
28. Cleanses perineum with toilet tissue or warm water and washcloth. Dries the perineum.			
29. Applies perineal pad if there is excessive drainage.			

Recommendation: Pass _____ Needs more practice _____

Student: _____   Date: _____

Instructor: _____   Date: _____

PROCEDURE CHECKLIST
Chapter 23: Inserting a Rectal Suppository

Check (✓) Yes or No

PROCEDURE STEPS	Yes	No	COMMENTS
1. Prepares and administers medications according to "Medication Guidelines: Steps to Follow for All Medications."			
2. Asks if the patient needs to defecate prior to the suppository insertion.			
3. Assists patient to Sims' position.			
4. If patient is uncooperative (e.g., confused, child) obtains help to immobilize the patient while inserting the suppository.			
5. Removes suppository wrapper and lubricates smooth end of the suppository and tip of the gloved index finger.			
6. Explains that there will be a cool feeling from the lubricant and a feeling of pressure during insertion.			
7. Uses nondominant hand to separate the buttocks.			
8. Asks patient to take deep breaths in and out through the mouth.			
9. Uses index finger of dominant hand, to gently insert suppository, lubricated smooth end first; or follows manufacturers' instructions.			
10. Does not force suppository during insertion.			
11. Pushes the suppository past the internal sphincter and along the rectal wall (about 4 inches or 10 cm in an adult; 2 inches or 5 cm for a child).			
12. If the client has difficulty retaining the suppository, after removing the finger from the anus, holds client's buttocks together for a few seconds or asks the patient to try to retain the suppository if he is able.			
13. Wipes anus with toilet tissue.			
14. Explains to patient the need to remain in side-lying position for 5 to 10 minutes.			
15. Leaves call light and bedpan within reach if suppository was a laxative.			

Recommendation: Pass _____ Needs more practice _____

Student: _____   Date: _____

Instructor: _____   Date: _____

PROCEDURE CHECKLIST
Chapter 23: Irrigating the Eyes

Check (✓) Yes or No

PROCEDURE STEPS	Yes	No	COMMENTS
1. Prepares and administers medications according to "Medication Guidelines: Steps to Follow for All Medications."			
2. Assists patient to low Fowler's position (if possible), with head tilted toward affected eye.			
3. Places towel and basin under patient's cheek.			
4. Checks pH by gently touching pH paper to secretions in the conjunctival sac (normal is approximately 7.1).			
5. Instills ocular anesthetic drops, if ordered or on protocol.			
6. Connects IV solution and tubing; primes the tubing.			
7. Holds IV tubing about 1 inch (2.5 cm) from the eye; does not touch the eye.			
8. Separates eyelids with thumb and index finger.			
9. Directs flow of solution over the eye from inner to outer canthus.			
10. Rechecks pH and continues to irrigate eye as needed.			

Recommendation: Pass _____ Needs more practice _____

Student: _____   Date: _____

Instructor: _____   Date: _____

PROCEDURE CHECKLIST
Chapter 23: Locating Intramuscular Injection Sites

Check (✓) Yes or No

PROCEDURE STEPS	Yes	No	COMMENTS
1. Palpates the landmarks and the muscle mass to ensure correct location and muscle adequacy.			
Deltoid Site			
2. Uses this site for small amounts of medication or when the ventrogluteal or vastus lateralis sites are contraindicated.			
3. Completely exposes the patient's upper arm, removing the garment if necessary.			
4. Locates the lower edge of the acromion process and goes two fingerbreadths down.			
5. Draws an imaginary line out from the axillary crease. The resulting inverted triangle is the deltoid site.			
6. An alternative approach is to place four fingerbreadths across the deltoid muscle with the top finger on the acromion process. The injection goes three fingerbreadths below the process.			
Dorsogluteal Site			
7. Uses this site only if no other sites are available.			
8. Has the patient lie prone.			
9. Locates the greater trochanter and the posterior superior iliac spine.			
10. Draws an imaginary line between the greater trochanter and the posterior superior iliac spine.			
11. In the middle of the line, goes superior (up) approximately 1 inch to locate the site.			
Rectus Femoris			
(Not a site of choice)			
12. Divides the top of the thigh from groin to the knee into thirds and identifies the middle third. Visualizes a rectangle in the middle of the anterior surface of the thigh. This is the location of the injection site.			
Vastus Lateralis			
13. Has patient assume supine or sitting position.			
14. Locates the greater trochanter and the lateral femoral condyle.			

PROCEDURE STEPS	Yes	No	COMMENTS
15. Places hands on patient's thigh with one hand against the greater trochanter and the edge of the other hand against the lateral femoral condyle.			
16. Visualizes a rectangle between the hands across the anterolateral thigh. The index fingers of the hands form the smaller ends of the rectangle. The long sides of the rectangle are formed by (a) drawing an imaginary line down the center of the anterior thigh, and (b) drawing another line along the side of the leg, halfway between the bed and the front of the thigh. This box marks the middle third of the anterolateral thigh, which is the injection site.			
Ventrogluteal Site			
17. Has patient assume a side-lying position, if possible.			
18. Locates the greater trochanter, anterior superior iliac spine, and the iliac crest.			
19. Places palm of hand on the greater trochanter, index finger on the anterior superior iliac spine, and the middle finger pointing toward the iliac crest. (Uses right hand on the patient's left hip; uses left hand on the patient's right hip.)			
20. The middle of the triangle between the middle and index fingers is the injection site.			

Recommendation: Pass _____ Needs more practice _____

Student: _____   Date: _____

Instructor: _____   Date: _____

PROCEDURE CHECKLIST
Chapter 23: Mixing Medications in One Syringe, Using a Prefilled Cartridge and Single-Dose Vial – For Intravenous Administration

Check (✓) Yes or No

PROCEDURE STEPS	Yes	No	COMMENTS
Refer to Procedure Checklist Chapter 23: Preparing and Drawing Up Medications from Ampules for handling ampules.			
Refer to Procedure Checklist Chapter 23: Preparing and Drawing Up Medications from Vials for handling vials.			
See Technique 23-4 in Volume 2 for measuring dosages when using filter needles.			
1. Prepares and administers medications according to "Medication Guidelines: Steps to Follow for All Medications."			
2. Checks compatibility of medications.			
3. Before beginning, determines total volume of all medications to be put in the syringe and whether that volume is appropriate for the administration site.			
4. When recapping sterile needles, uses a needle capping device or approved one-handed technique that has a low risk of contaminating the sterile needle.			
5. Holds syringe at eye level when checking and rechecking medication dose.			
6. Maintains sterility of needles and medication throughout the procedure.			
7. Wipes top of vial with alcohol prep pad, according to agency procedure.			
8. Assembles prefilled cartridge and holder according to manufacturer's directions.			
NOTE: If prefilled cartridge is not large enough to hold both medications, follow Technique 23-2 in Volume 2 to transfer cartridge contents to a second syringe with a removable needle. If cartridge will hold both medications, uses the following steps.			
9. Places needle (or access device) cap on opened, sterile alcohol wipe package.			
10. Holds syringe vertically and at eye level to expel air and read dose. If necessary to eject some medication, moves syringe to horizontal to do so.			
11. Draws up an amount of air equal to the amount of medication to be withdrawn from the vial.			

PROCEDURE STEPS	Yes	No	COMMENTS

12. Maintaining sterility, inserts needle or needleless device into vial without coring:
 	
    a. Places the tip of the needle or needleless device in the middle of the rubber top of the vial with the bevel up at a 45°–60° angle.
    b. While pushing the needle or needleless device into the rubber top, gradually brings the needle upright to a 90° angle.			

13. With bevel of the needle above the fluid line, injects the air in the syringe into the air in the vial, not into the fluid. Is careful not to eject any medication from the cartridge into the vial.			
14. Inverts vial, keeps needle in the medication, and slowly withdraws medication. Takes care not to draw in more than the amount needed (e.g., if 1 mL of each drug is ordered, the plunger should be at 2 mL at the end of this step). Keeps index finger on the flange of the syringe to prevent it being forced back by pressure.			
15. Keeping needle in vial, expels air bubbles from syringe back into the vial. a. Carefully stabilizes the vial and syringe and firmly tap the syringe below the air bubbles.			
b. When the air bubbles are at the hub of the syringe, makes sure the syringe is vertical, and pushes the air back into the vial.			
c. Withdraws additional medication if necessary to obtain the correct dose.			
16. Withdraws needle or vial access device from vial at a 90° angle.			
17. If combined medications in the syringe exceed the total amount initially calculated, recognizes error, discards medication, and begins again.			
18. Recaps needle.			

Recommendation: Pass _____ Needs more practice _____

Student: _____   Date: _____

Instructor: _____   Date: _____

PROCEDURE CHECKLIST
Chapter 23: Mixing Medications in One Syringe, Using One Ampule and Vial

Check (✓) Yes or No

PROCEDURE STEPS	Yes	No	COMMENTS
1. Prepares and administers medications according to "Medication Guidelines: Steps to Follow for All Medications."			
2. Checks compatibility of medications.			
3. Before beginning, determines total volume of all medications to be put in the syringe and whether that volume is appropriate for the administration site.			
4. When recapping sterile needles, uses a needle capping device or approved one-handed technique that has a low risk of contaminating the sterile needle (see Procedure Checklist Chapter 23: Recapping Needles Using One-Handed Technique).			
5. Recaps needles throughout, using a needle capping device or approved one-handed technique that has a low risk of contaminating the sterile needle.			
6. Maintains sterility of needles and medication throughout the procedure.			
7. Cleanses tops of vial with alcohol prep pad (according to agency procedure).			
8. Withdraws from the vial first. Places needle cap on opened sterile alcohol wipe wrapper (sterile field).			
9. Draws up same amount of air into syringe as the total ordered dose for the medication in the vial.			
10. Keeping the tip of the needle (or needleless device) above the medication, injects the amount of air equal to the volume of drug to be withdrawn from the vial.			
11. Without removing the needle (or needleless device) from the vial, inverts the vial and withdraws the ordered amount of medication.			
12. Using correct technique, expels any air bubbles and measures dose at eye level. Removes air bubbles, rechecks dosage, and withdraws more or ejects drug as needed (see Procedure Checklist Chapter 23: Mixing Medications in One Syringe, Using Two Vials).			
13. Recaps and removes needle, places on opened, sterile alcohol wipe.			
14. Attaches a filter needle to the syringe (if not done at step 8).			

PROCEDURE STEPS	Yes	No	COMMENTS
15. Flicks or taps the top of the ampule to remove medication trapped in the top of the ampule. Alternatively, shakes the ampule by quickly turning and "snapping" the wrist.			
16. Uses ampule snapper, or wraps 2×2 gauze pad or unwrapped alcohol wipe around neck of the ampule; using dominant hand, snaps off the top.			
17. Breaks ampule top away from the body.			
18. Does not touch the neck of the ampule with the needle while withdrawing medication.			
19. Uses one of the following techniques to withdraw correct amount of medication (filter needle should still be on the syringe): a. Inverts ampule, places needle tip in liquid, and withdraw all of medication. Does not insert needle through the medication into the air at the top of the inverted ampule b. Alternatively, tips ampule, places needle in liquid, and withdraws medication. Repositions ampule so that needle tip remains in the liquid.			
20. When drawing up second medication (from ampule) does not draw excess medication into the syringe. If this occurs, recognizes error, discards, and repeats procedure.			
21. Draws enough air into the syringe to clear the filter needle (see Technique 23-4 in Volume 2), about 0.2 mL.			
22. Recaps and removes filter needle and discards it in the sharps container.			
23. Attaches the "saved" (or new) sterile needle for administration.			
24. Holds syringe vertically and checks exact medication dose at eye level. (Plunger should be at the "total combined dose + 0.2 mL" line). Alternatively, ejects the air (" drop to the top") and checks that the total combined dose is correct, with no air in the syringe.			
25. If total dose is not exact, discards medication and begins again.			
26. Recaps administration needle, using accepted technique.			

Recommendation: Pass _____ Needs more practice _____

Student: _____   Date: _____

Instructor: _____   Date: _____

PROCEDURE CHECKLIST
Chapter 23: Mixing Medications in One Syringe, Using Two Vials

Check (✓) Yes or No

PROCEDURE STEPS	Yes	No	COMMENTS
1. Prepares and administers medications according to "Medication Guidelines: Steps to Follow for All Medications."			
2. Checks compatibility of medications.			
3. Before beginning, determines total volume of all medications to be put in the syringe and whether that volume is appropriate for the administration site.			
4. Recaps needles throughout, using a needle capping device or approved one-handed technique that has a low risk of contaminating the sterile needle (see Procedure Checklist Chapter 23: Recapping Needles Using One-Handed Technique).			
5. Maintains sterility of needles and medication throughout the procedure.			
6. Avoids contaminating a multi-dose vial with a second medication.			
7. Cleanses tops of vials with alcohol prep pad (according to agency procedure).			
8. Places needle cap on opened, sterile alcohol wipe.			
9. Draws up same amount of air into syringe as the total medication doses for both vials (e.g., if the order is for 0.5 mL for Vial A and 1 mL for Vial B, draws up 1.5 mL of air).			

10. Maintaining sterility, inserts needle or vial access cannula into vial without coring (or uses a filter needle):
    a. Places the tip of the needle or vial access cannula in the middle of the rubber top of the vial with the bevel up at a 45°–60° angle.
    b. While pushing the needle or vial cannula device into the rubber top, gradually brings the needle upright to a 90° angle.			

11. Keeping the tip of the needle (or vial access device) above the medication, injects amount of air equal to the volume of drug to be withdrawn from the first vial (e.g., 0.5 mL for Vial A in step 9; then injects the rest of the air into the second vial.			
NOTE: If one vial is a multi-dose vial, injects air into the multiple-dose vial first.			

PROCEDURE STEPS	Yes	No	COMMENTS
NOTE: If mixing two types of insulin, puts air into the regular insulin last. Refer to Technique 23-8, in Volume 2, for mixing two types of insulin.			
12a. Without removing the needle (or access device) from the second vial, inverts the vial and withdraws the ordered amount of medication.			
12b. Using correct technique expels any air bubbles and measures dose at eye level. (See Procedure Checklist Chapter 23: Preparing and Drawing Up Medications from Vials.)			
12c. Removes needle from vial and pulls back on the plunger enough to pull all medication out of the needle (or access device) into the syringe.			
12d. Reads dose at eye level; holds syringe vertically to eject all air; tips syringe horizontally if any medication must be ejected.			
13a. Inserts needle into first vial, inverts, and withdraws the exact ordered amount of medication, holding syringe vertical (when finished, the plunger should be at the line for the total/combined dose.			
13b. Keeps index finger on the flange of the syringe to prevent it being forced back by pressure. Does not draw excess medication into the syringe.			
13c. If excess medication is inadvertently drawn into syringe, recognizes error, discards the medication in the syringe, and starts over. (The "total" amount calculated initially should be in the syringe.)			
14. If a filter needle or VAD was used, draws air into syringe to clear medication from needle and proceeds according to Technique 23-4 in Volume 2.			
15. Removes needle from vial and recaps needle, using needle capping device or approved one-handed scoop method.			
16. Places a new sterile needle on the syringe to be used to give the injection.			
17. Next holds syringe vertically and re-checks the dosage at eye level.			

Recommendation: Pass _____ Needs more practice _____

Student: _____ Date: _____

Instructor: _____ Date: _____

PROCEDURE CHECKLIST
Chapter 23: Preparing and Drawing Up Medications from Ampules

Check (✓) Yes or No

PROCEDURE STEPS	Yes	No	COMMENTS
1. Prepares and administers medications according to "Medication Guidelines: Steps to Follow for All Medications."			
2. Recaps needles throughout, using a needle capping device or approved one-handed technique that has a low risk of contaminating the sterile needle (see Procedure Checklist Chapter 23: Recapping Needles Using One-Handed Technique).			
3. Flicks or taps the top of the ampule to remove medication trapped in the top of the ampule. Alternatively, shakes the ampule by quickly turning and "snapping" the wrist.			
4. Uses ampule snapper, or wraps 2×2 gauze pad or unwrapped alcohol wipe around neck of the ampule; using dominant hand, snaps off the top.			
5. Breaks ampule top away from the body.			
6. Attaches filter needle (or filter straw) to a syringe. If syringe has a needle in place, removes both the needle and the cap and places on a sterile surface (e.g., a newly unwrapped alcohol pad still in the open wrapper), then attaches filter needle.			
7. Does not touch the neck of the ampule with the needle while withdrawing medication.			

8. Uses one of the following techniques to withdraw medication:
  a. Inverts ampule, places needle tip in liquid, and withdraws all of medication. Does not insert needle through the medication into the air at the top of the inverted ampule.
  b. Alternatively, tips ampule, places needle in liquid, and withdraws all medication. Repositions ampule so that needle tip remains in the liquid.			

9. Draws up exact amount of medication.			
10. If necessary to eject medication after ejecting air, tips the syringe horizontal to do so.			

PROCEDURE STEPS	Yes	No	COMMENTS
11. Holds syringe vertically and draws 0.2 mL of air into the syringe. Measures exact medication dose (draws back plunger to the "dose + 0.2 mL" line).			
12. Removes filter needle and reattaches the "saved" (or other sterile) needle for administration.			
13. Ejects the 0.2 mL of air, and checks the dose again. (If giving an irritating medication such as parenteral iron, omit this step.)			
14. Disposes of top and bottom of ampule and filter needle in a sharps container.			

Recommendation: Pass _____ Needs more practice _____

Student: _____   Date: _____

Instructor: _____   Date: _____

PROCEDURE CHECKLIST
Chapter 23: Preparing and Drawing Up Medications from Vials

Check (✓) Yes or No

PROCEDURE STEPS	Yes	No	COMMENTS
1. Prepares and administers medications according to "Medication Guidelines: Steps to Follow for All Medications."			
2. Maintains sterility during all steps.			
3. Recaps needles throughout, using a needle capping device or approved one-handed technique that has a low risk of contaminating the sterile needle (see Procedure Checklist Chapter 23: Recapping Needles Using One-Handed Technique).			
4. Mixes solution in vial, if needed, by gently rolling between hands.			
5. If using a multi-dose vial, places it on flat work surface and thoroughly cleans rubber top of vial with alcohol prep pad.			
a. Uncaps needle without touching needle tip or shaft; places needle cap on a clean surface or holds open side out between two fingers of nondominant hand. b. Or if using a vial access device, attaches the device to the syringe and removes the cap, maintaining sterility.			
6. Draws air into the syringe equal to the amount of medication to be withdrawn.			
7. Maintaining sterility, inserts needle or vial access cannula into vial without coring (or uses a filter needle): a. Places the tip of the needle or vial access cannula in the middle of the rubber top of the vial with the bevel up at a 45°–60° angle. b. While pushing the needle or vial cannula device into the rubber top, gradually brings the needle upright to a 90° angle.			
8. With bevel of the needle above the fluid line, injects the air in the syringe into the air in the vial, not into the fluid.			
9. Inverts vial, keeps needle or vial access device in the medication, and slowly withdraws medication.			

PROCEDURE STEPS	Yes	No	COMMENTS
10. Keeping needle or vial access device in vial, expels air bubbles from syringe back into the vial.			
a. Carefully stabilizes the vial and syringe and firmly taps the syringe below the air bubbles.			
b. When the air bubbles are at the hub of the syringe, makes sure the syringe is vertical, and pushes the air back into the vial.			
c. Withdraws additional medication if necessary to obtain the correct dose.			
11. When the dose is correct, withdraws needle or vial access device from vial at a 90° angle.			
12. Holds syringe upright at eye level when checking and rechecking medication dose.			
13. If using a filter needle, draws 0.2 mL of air into the syringe, measures medication, and ejects air., as directed in Procedure Checklist Chapter 23: Preparing and Drawing Up Medications from Ampules.			
14. Recaps needle or injection cannula using needle recapping device or an approved one-handed method.			
15. If administering an irritating medication or if a vial access device or filter needle was used to draw up medication, changes the needle prior to administration.			
16. If needle must be changed, follows these steps: a. Holds syringe vertically and draws 0.2 mL of air into the syringe. Holds at eye level and re-checks measured dose. b. Removes filter (or other) needle and reattaches the "saved" (or other sterile) needle for administration c. Measures exact medication dose. Holds syringe vertically to expel all the air. d. If necessary to eject medication after ejecting air, tips the syringe horizontal to do so.			
17. Disposes of vial and filter needle(s) in a sharps container.			

Recommendation: Pass _____ Needs more practice _____

Student: _____   Date: _____

Instructor: _____   Date: _____

Check (✓) Yes or No

PROCEDURE STEPS	Yes	No	COMMENTS
Recapping Contaminated Needles			
1. Recaps a contaminated needle only if it must be done for personal or patient safety.			
2. Does not place nondominant hand near the needle cap when recapping or engaging the safety mechanism.			
3. If safety needle is being used, engages safety mechanism to cover needle; or, if available, places needle cap in mechanical recapping device.			

4. If recapping devices are not available, recaps using the following one-handed scoop technique:
  a. Places the needle cover on flat surface.
  b. Then, holding syringe in the dominant hand, scoops the needle cap onto the needle.
  c. Tips syringe vertically to slide cover over needle.
  d. Does not hold onto the needle cap with nondominant hand while scooping—keeps nondominant hand well away from needle cap.
  e. Secures the needle cap by grasping it near the hub.			

Recapping Sterile Needles			
5. Does not contaminate the sterile needle.			

6. Uses one of the following techniques correctly:
  a. Places needle cap into medication cup with open end facing up. Then inserts the sterile needle into the cap, keeping free hand well away from the cup.
  b. Or places the cap on a clean surface so the end of the needle cap protrudes out over the edge of the counter or shelf. Scoops cap up with the needle, keeping the free hand well away from the needle and cap while recapping.
  c. Or, if syringe is packaged in hard plastic, stands the hard package on its larger end. Inserts the needle cap in the small (top) end; then, holding the syringe in dominant hand, inserts the needle downward and firmly into the cap.
  d. Or, places the needle cap on a sterile surface, such as an open alcohol prep pad, and uses a one-handed scoop technique. (This is not a preferred method because the risk of touching the needle to an nonsterile surface is high, especially for novices.)			

PROCEDURE STEPS	Yes	No	COMMENTS

Recommendation: Pass _____ Needs more practice _____

Student: _____   Date: _____

Instructor: _____   Date: _____

PROCEDURE CHECKLIST
Chapter 23: Using a Piggyback Set

Check (✓) Yes or No

PROCEDURE STEPS	Yes	No	COMMENTS
1. Prepares and administers medications according to "Medication Guidelines: Steps to Follow for All Medications."			
2. Draws up the medication and injects it into the piggyback solution (see Procedure Checklist Chapter 23: Adding Medications to Intravenous Fluids). This step is not necessary if the medication comes premixed from the pharmacy.			
3. Chooses the correct tubing (secondary tubing is long; piggyback tubing is short).			
4. Attaches the piggyback tubing to the medication bag without touching the spike.			
5. Squeezes the drip chamber, filling it 1/3 to 1/2 full.			
6a. Opens the clamp and primes the tubing, holding the end of the tubing lower than the bag of fluid.			
6b. Does not let more than one drop of fluid escape from the end of the tubing.			
6c. Closes the clamp.			
6d. Cleanses the primary "Y" port.			
7. Alternatively, instead of Step 6, "back-flushes" the piggyback line.			
a. Clamps the piggyback tubing.			
b. Cleanses the primary "Y" port.			
c. Attaches the piggyback tubing with a needleless system.			
d. Opens clamp on piggyback tubing and lowers the bag below the primary bag to allow fluid to flow up the piggyback line.			
e. Once the air is out of the piggyback line, clamps the piggyback tubing.			
8a. Labels the bag with date, medication, dosage, and initials of person preparing medication. 8b. Labels the tubing with time, date, and initials of person preparing.			
9. Hangs the piggyback container on the IV pole. Lowers the primary IV container to hang below the level of the piggyback IV.			
10. Opens the clamp of piggyback line (if there is a roller clamp, opens it completely).			

PROCEDURE STEPS	Yes	No	COMMENTS
11. Regulates the drip rate with the roller clamp on the primary line. Regulates to the prescribed infusion rate for the medication.			
12. At the end of the infusion, clamps the piggyback tubing, moves the primary tubing back to its original height.			
13. Uses the roller clamp to reset the primary bag to its correct infusion rate.			

Recommendation: Pass _____ Needs more practice _____

Student: _____   Date: _____

Instructor: _____   Date: _____

PROCEDURE CHECKLIST
Chapter 23: Using a Tandem (Secondary) Set

Check (✓) Yes or No

PROCEDURE STEPS	Yes	No	COMMENTS
1. Prepares and administers medications according to "Medication Guidelines: Steps to Follow for All Medications."			
2. Draws up the medication and injects it into the tandem (secondary) solution (see Procedure Checklist Chapter 23: Adding Medications to Intravenous Fluids). This step is not necessary if the medication comes premixed from the pharmacy.			
3. Chooses the correct tubing (secondary tubing is long; piggyback tubing is short).			
4. Squeezes the drip chamber, filling it 1/3 to 1/2 full.			
5a. Opens the clamp and primes the tubing, holding the end of the tubing lower than the bag of fluid.			
5b. Does not let more than one drop of fluid escape from the end of the tubing.			
5c. Closes the clamp.			
5d. Cleanses the primary "Y" port.			
6. Alternatively, instead of Step 5, "back-flushes" the tandem line, after doing Steps 7 through 9. See Step 10 for "back-flushing."			
7. Labels the bag with date, medication, dosage, and initials of person preparing medication.			
8. Labels the tubing with time, date, and initials of person preparing.			
9. Hangs the secondary bag at same height as primary bag.			
10. If not using Step 5, "back-flushes" the tandem line: a. Clamps the tandem tubing.			
b. Cleanses the secondary port (the one nearest the patient) with an antimicrobial swab.			
c. Attaches tandem tubing with needleless system.			
d. Opens clamp on secondary tubing and lowers the bag below the primary bag to allow fluid to flow up and prime the secondary line.			
e. Once the line is primed, clamps the secondary tubing.			
11. Runs both the secondary and primary bags simultaneously. Unclamps secondary tubing and regulates the secondary infusion at the prescribed rate, using the roller clamp on the secondary line.			

PROCEDURE STEPS	Yes	No	COMMENTS
12. Also reverifies the primary bag rate.			
13. At the end of the infusion, clamps the secondary tubing.			
14. Rechecks the flow rate of the primary bag.			
15. Disposes of used supplies safely and according to agency procedures.			

Recommendation: Pass _____ Needs more practice _____

Student: _____   Date: _____

Instructor: _____   Date: _____

PROCEDURE CHECKLIST
Chapter 23: Using a Volume-Control Administration Set (e.g., Buretrol, Volutrol, Soluset)

Check (✓) Yes or No

PROCEDURE STEPS	Yes	No	COMMENTS
1. Prepares and administers medications according to "Medication Guidelines: Steps to Follow for All Medications."			
2. Prepares volume-control set tubing.			
a. Closes both upper and lower clamps on tubing.			
b. Opens clamp of air vent on volume-control chamber (see Procedure Checklist Chapter 36: Initiating a Peripheral Intravenous Infusion).			
c. Maintaining sterile procedure, attaches administration spike of the volume-control set to the primary IV bag.			
d. Fills the volume-control chamber with the desired amount of IV solution by opening the clamp between the IV bag and the volume-control chamber. When the correct amount of solution is in the chamber, closes the clamp.			
e. Primes the rest of the tubing by pinching the drip chamber (of the volume-control set), filling it half full, opening the clamp below the chamber, and running the IV fluid until all the air has been expelled.			
f. Rechecks volume and if needed adds additional fluid to desired amount.			
3. Connects end of the volume-control IV line to the patient's IV site. Attaches directly to IV catheter, to extension tubing, or to injection port closest to patient. If using injection port, cleanses port with alcohol or other antiseptic wipe.			
4. Cleanses the injection port on the volume-control chamber.			
5. Attaches the medication syringe (preferably with a blunt, needleless device), and injects the medication into the solution in the chamber.			
6. If using a needle, disposes of syringe and needle.			
7. Gently rotates the chamber to mix the medication in the IV solution.			
8. Opens the lower clamp and starts the infusion at the correct flow rate.			

PROCEDURE STEPS	Yes	No	COMMENTS
9. Labels the volume-control chamber with the date, time, medication, and doses added, and initials according to agency policy.			
10. When the medication has finished infusing, adds a small amount of the primary fluid to the chamber and flushes the tubing. Uses two times the volume in the dead space of the tubing as the flush volume (check tubing package for amount).			

Recommendation: Pass _____ Needs more practice _____

Student: _____   Date: _____

Instructor: _____   Date: _____

PROCEDURE CHECKLIST
Chapter 26: Administering Feedings Through Gastric and Enteric Tubes

Check (✓) Yes or No

PROCEDURE STEPS	Yes	No	COMMENTS
1. Determines type of feeding, rate of infusion, and frequency of feeding.			
2. Checks expiration date of the feeding formula.			
3. Warms formula to room temperature (for continuous feedings, keeps formula cool but not cold).			
4. Shakes the feeding formula to mix well.			
5. Prepares equipment for administration. **For Open System with Feeding Bag:** 　a. Fills disposable tube feeding (TF) bag with a 4- to 6-hour supply of formula; primes the tubing. 　b. Labels TF bag with date, time, formula type, and rate. 　c. Hangs the TF bag on an IV pole. **For Open System with Syringe:** a. Prepares the syringe by removing the plunger. **For Closed System with Prefilled Bottle with Drip Chamber:** 　a. Attaches administration set to prefilled bottle and primes tubing. 　b. Hangs the prefilled bottle on an IV pole.			
6. Elevates head of the bed at least 30°.			
7. Places a linen saver pad under the connection end of the feeding tube.			
8. Dons procedure gloves.			
9. For the first feeding, verifies tube placement by: 　a. Aspirating stomach contents and measuring pH. 　b. Confirms findings by asking the patient to speak. 　c. For NG and NE tubes, but not for gastrostomy or jejunostomy tubes, can also confirm by injecting air into the tube and auscultating.			
10. For subsequent feedings, aspirates and measures gastric residual (except for jejunostomy tubes). 　a. Connects syringe to the proximal end of the feeding tube. 　b. Measures volume of aspirated contents using syringe (if volume is more than 60 mL, uses graduated container).			

PROCEDURE STEPS	Yes	No	COMMENTS
c. Reinstills aspirate unless the volume is more than the formula flow rate for 1 hour (or alternatively, a total of 150 mL). If the aspirate volume is more than the formula flow rate for 1 hour or 150 mL, notifies the physician.			
11. Flushes the feeding tube with 30 mL of tap water.			
Beginning the Feeding			
12. **If Using an Infusion Pump:** a. Threads the administration tubing through the infusion pump according to manufacturer's instructions.			
b. Clamps or pinches off the end of the feeding tube to prevent air from entering the tube.			
c. If a connector is needed, attaches it to the proximal end of the feeding tube. Connects the distal end of the administration tubing to the connector. If no connector is needed, attaches the distal end of the administration tubing to the proximal end of the feeding tube.			
d. Turns on infusion pump; sets pump with correct infusion rate and volume.			
13. **If Using Open System and Syringe:** a. Clamps or pinches off the end of the feeding tube.			
b. Attaches the syringe to the proximal end of the feeding tube.			
c. Fills the syringe with the prescribed amount of formula.			
d. Releases tube clamp or "pinch," and elevates the syringe. Does not elevate syringe >18 inches above the tube insertion site.			
e. Allows feeding to flow slowly (if too fast, lowers the syringe).			
f. When the syringe is 3/4 empty, clamps tube or holds it above the level of the stomach; refills syringe; unclamps and continues feeding until prescribed amount is administered.			
14. **Using a Closed System with a Prefilled Bottle with a Drip Chamber (No Infusion Pump):** a. If connector is needed, attaches to the proximal end of the feeding tube. Connects distal end of administration tubing to the connector. If no connector is needed, attaches distal end of the administration tube to the proximal end of the feeding tube.			

PROCEDURE STEPS	Yes	No	COMMENTS
b. Opens the roller clamp on the administration tubing and regulates the flow to the ordered rate.			
Ending Feeding			
14. When feeding is infused, clamps or pinches off the proximal end of the feeding tube. If an infusion pump was used, turns off the pump before pinching off the proximal end of the feeding tube.			
15. Disconnects the syringe or administration tubing from the feeding tube. Flushes the feeding tube with 30 mL of tap water. If administering a continuous feeding, flushes the tube with the prescribed amount of water (typically 50 to 100 mL) every 4 to 6 hours.			
16. Caps the proximal end of the feeding tube.			
17. Changes tube feeding bag, administration set, and syringes every 24 hours (or according to agency policy).			
18. Keeps head of patient's bed elevated at least 30° for 1 hour after administering the feeding.			
19. **Procedure Variation: Gastrostomy or Jejunostomy Tubes:** Cleans insertion site daily with soap and water. A small, precut, gauze dressing may be applied to site.			
20. **Procedure Variation for Cuffed Tracheostomy Tube:** If the patient has a cuffed tracheostomy tube, inflate the cuff before administering the feeding and keep the cuff inflated at for least 15 minutes afterward.			

Recommendation: Pass _____ Needs more practice _____

Student: _____   Date: _____

Instructor: _____   Date: _____

PROCEDURE CHECKLIST
Chapter 26 - Checking Fingerstick (Capillary) Blood Glucose Levels

Check (✓) Yes or No

PROCEDURE STEPS	Yes	No	COMMENTS
1. Has the patient wash her hands with soap and warm water, if she is able.			
2. If patient is in bed, assists to semi-Fowler's position if possible.			
3. Turns on the glucose meter. Calibrates according to manufacturer's instructions.			
4. Checks expiration date on the container or reagent strips.			
5. Removes a reagent strip, then tightly seals container.			
6. Checks that the reagent strip is the correct type for the monitor being used.			
7. Dons procedure gloves.			
8. Selects a puncture site on the lateral aspect of a finger (heel or great toe for an infant).			
9. Positions the finger in a dependent position and massages toward the fingertip.			
10. For infants, older adults, and people with poor circulation, places a warm cloth on the site for about 10 minutes before obtaining the blood sample.			
11. Cleanses the site with an antiseptic pad, or according to facility policy, and dries it with a gauze pad.			
12a. Engages the sterile lancet and removes the cover.			
12b. Places the back of the hand on the table, or otherwise secures the finger so it does not move when pricked.			
12c. Positions the sterile lancet firmly against the skin, perpendicular to the puncture site. Pushes the release switch, allowing the needle to pierce the skin.			
13. If there is no injector, uses a darting motion to prick the site with the lancet.			
14. Lightly squeezes the patient's finger above the puncture site until a droplet of blood has collected.			
15. Wipes away the first drop and squeezes again to form another droplet.			

PROCEDURE STEPS	Yes	No	COMMENTS
16. Places reagent strip test patch close to the drop of blood. Allows contact between the drop of blood and the test patch until blood covers the entire patch. Does not "smear" the blood over the reagent strip.			
17. Allows the blood sample to remain in contact with the reagent strip for the amount of time specified by the manufacturer.			
18. Using a gauze pad, gently applies pressure to the puncture site.			
19. Places the reagent strip into the glucose meter. (Some manufacturer's instructions require you to first wipe the reagent strip with a cotton ball so that no blood remains on the test patch. Follows individual manufacturer instructions.)			
20. After the meter signals, reads the blood glucose level indicated on the digital display.			
21. Turns off the meter and disposes of the reagent strip, cotton ball, gauze pad, paper towel, alcohol pad, and lancet in the proper containers.			
22. Removes the procedure gloves and disposes of them in the proper container.			

Recommendation: Pass _____ Needs more practice _____

Student: _____   Date: _____

Instructor: _____   Date: _____

Check (✓) Yes or No

PROCEDURE STEPS	Yes	No	COMMENTS
1. Prepares the tube. a. Plastic tube: Places in basin of warm water for 10 minutes. b. Rubber tube: Places in basin of ice for 10 minutes. c. Small-bore tube: Inserts stylet or guidewire and secures into position according to agency policy. (Small bore tubes may come with the guidewire in them. Leaves the wire in place until tube is positioned and placement checked on x-ray. Once wire is removed, does not reinsert it.)			
2. Assists patient into a high Fowler's position. **Variations:** a. If the patient is comatose, places the patient into a semi-Fowler's position. Has a coworker help position the patient's head for insertion. b. If the patient is confused and combative, asks a coworker to assist with insertion.			
3. Measures tube length correctly. a. <u>Nasogastric tube</u>: Measures from the tip of the nose to the earlobe, and from the earlobe to the xiphoid process. Marks the length with tape or indelible ink on the NG tube. b. <u>Nasoenteric tube</u>: Adds 8–10 cm (3–4 inches) to NG measurement and marks with tape.			
4. Drapes a linen saver pad over the patient's chest and hands him an emesis basin.			
5. Cuts a 4-inch (10 cm) piece of hypoallergenic tape.			
6. Dons procedure gloves, if not done previously.			
7. Lubricates the distal 4 inches (10 cm) of the tube with a water-soluble lubricant.			
8. If the patient is awake, alert, and able to swallow, hands him a glass of water with a straw.			
9a. Gently inserts the tip of the tube into the nostril. Has the patient hyperextend his neck and advances the tube slowly, aiming downward and toward the ear.			

PROCEDURE STEPS	Yes	No	COMMENTS
9b. If resistance is felt when the tube reaches the nasopharynx, uses gentle pressure, but does not force the tube to advance.			
9c. Provides tissues if the patient's eyes tear.			
10. After the tube passes through the nasopharynx, has the patient flex his head toward the chest.			
11. Rotates the tube 180°.			
12. Directs patient to sip and swallow the water while slowly advancing the tube.			
13. Advances tube 2–4 inches (5–10 cm) with each swallow until marked length is reached.			
14a. If patient gags, stops advancing the tube and has patient take deep breaths and drink a few sips of water.			
14b. If gagging continues, uses a tongue blade and penlight to check tube position in the back of the throat.			
14c. If the tube is coiled in the back of the throat, the patient coughs excessively during insertion, the tube does not advance with each swallow, or the patient develops respiratory distress, withdraws the tube and allow the patient to rest before reinserting.			
14d. **Variation: To Advance the Tube Into the Duodenum:** After the tube is in the stomach, positions patient on his right side; advances the tube 5 to 7.5 cm (2 to 3 inches) hourly, over several hours (up to 24 hours) until radiography confirms placement.			
15. When tube is in place, secures it temporarily with one piece of tape so it does not move while confirming placement.			
16. Verifies tube placement at the bedside by: a. Aspirating stomach contents and measuring pH. b. Confirms "a" by injecting air into the NG tube and auscultating, or asking patient to speak. (See Technique 28-4 in Volume 2.)			
17. After confirming placement, secures tube with tape or a tube fixation device. **Tape:** a. Applies skin adhesive to patient's nose and allows it to dry.			
b. Removes gloves and tears one end of the hypoallergenic tape lengthwise for 2 inches (5 cm)			

PROCEDURE STEPS	Yes	No	COMMENTS
c. Applies the intact end of the tape to the patient's nose.			
d. Wraps the 2-inch (5 cm) strips around the tube where it exits the nose.			
e. Alternatively, uses 1-inch tape; applies one end to patient's nose, wraps the middle around the tube, and secures the other end to the opposite side of the nose.			
Alternative: Uses Fixation device: Places the wide end of the pad over the bridge of the nose; positions the connector around the tube where it exits the nose.			
18. Ties a slipknot around the tube with a rubber band. Secures the rubber band (or tape) to the patient's gown with a safety pin.			

Recommendation: Pass _____ Needs more practice _____

Student: _____ Date: _____

Instructor: _____ Date: _____

PROCEDURE CHECKLIST
Chapter 26: Removing a Nasogastric or Nasoenteric Tube

Check (✓) Yes or No

PROCEDURE STEPS	Yes	No	COMMENTS
1. Assists the patient to a sitting or high Fowler's position.			
2. Places disposable plastic bag on the bed or within reach.			
3. Drapes a linen-saver pad across the patient's chest.			
4. Dons procedure gloves.			
5. Attaches the a 60 mL syringe to the proximal end of the tube and flushes with 10 mL of air.			
6. Unpins the tube from the patient's gown and then untapes the tube from the patient's nose.			
7. Pinches the proximal end of the tube.			
8. Asks patient to hold his breath.			
9. Quickly and gently withdraws the tube and places it in the plastic bag.			
10. Hands the patient a tissue.			
11. Provides mouth care.			
12. Removes gloves and disposes of gloves and tube in the nearest receptacle, according to facility policy.			

Recommendation: Pass _____ Needs more practice _____

Student: _____ Date: _____

Instructor: _____ Date: _____

PROCEDURE CHECKLIST
Chapter 27: Applying an External (Condom) Catheter

Check (✓) Yes or No

PROCEDURE STEPS	Yes	No	COMMENTS
1. Assesses skin of the penis.			
2. Uses clean technique throughout (medical asepsis).			
3. Prepares the leg bag or bedside drainage bag for attachment to the condom catheter by removing it from the packaging and placing the end of the connecting tubing near the perineal area.			
4. Rolls the condom catheter outward onto itself to prepare for rolling up and onto the penis.			
5. Places the patient in the supine position. For patients whose respiratory efforts may be impaired, raises the head of the bed to 30°.			
6. Folds down the bedcovers to expose the genitalia and drapes the patient, using the bath blanket.			
7. Washes hands.			
8. Dons clean procedure gloves.			
9. Gently cleanses the penis with soap and water. Rinses and dries thoroughly.			
10. If the penis is uncircumcised, retracts the foreskin, cleanses the glans and replaces the foreskin.			
11. Clips excess hair along the shaft of the penis, unless contraindicated by policy or patient's condition.			
12. Washes hands; changes procedure gloves.			
13. Measures circumference of the penis. Ensures catheter is appropriately sized.			
14. Applies skin prep (according to agency policy) and allows it to dry. (Some condom catheters require that a special adhesive strip be placed onto the penis prior to application of the condom; follows manufacturer's directions.)			
15. Holding penis in nondominant hand, with dominant hand places the condom at the end of the penis and slowly unrolls it up and along the shaft.			
16. Leaves 1 to 2 inches (2.5 to 5 cm) between the end of the penis and the drainage tube on the catheter.			
17. Secures condom catheter in place on the penis.			

PROCEDURE STEPS	Yes	No	COMMENTS
a. Ensures that the condom is not twisted.			
b. For condom catheters with internal adhesive, gently grasps the penis and compresses so that the entire shaft comes in contact with the condom.			
c. For condom catheters with external adhesives strips, wraps the strip around the outside of the condom in a spiral direction, taking care not to overlap the ends.			
18. Does not use regular bandage tape to hold a condom catheter in place.			
19. Assesses the proximal end of the condom catheter. If there is a large portion of the condom still rolled above the adhesive strip, clips the roll.			
20. Attaches the tube end of the condom catheter to a drainage system, making sure there are no kinks in the tubing.			
21. Secures the drainage tubing to the patient's thigh using tape or a commercial leg strap (follow facility protocol)..			
22. Covers the patient.			
23. Removes gloves and washes the hands.			

Recommendation: Pass _____ Needs more practice _____

Student: _____   Date: _____

Instructor: _____   Date: _____

PROCEDURE CHECKLIST
Chapter 27: Collecting a Clean-Catch Urine Specimen

Check (✓) Yes or No

PROCEDURE STEPS	Yes	No	COMMENTS
NOTE: *If patient is can do self care, instructs patient in the following steps. If not, performs them for the patient.*			
1. Assists patient to toilet, commode, or onto bedpan.			
2. Opens prepackaged kit, if available, and removes contents.			
3. Washes hands and dons clean procedure gloves.			
4. Instructs patient to cleanse around the urinary meatus if able; if not able, performs cleansing.			
Female Patients			
5. Asks patient to spread her legs; washes perineal area with warm water and mild soap.			
6. Opens the antiseptic towelette in the prepackaged kit. If there is no kit, pours antiseptic solution over cotton balls.			
7. Cleanses perineal area in a front-to-back direction; cleanses over the urinary meatus.			
8. Cleans the perineal area at least twice.			
9. Uses each towelette area or each cotton ball only once.			
Male Patients			
10. If penis is uncircumcised, retracts the foreskin back from the end of the penis.			
11. Uses towelette from the prepackaged kit or pours antiseptic solution over cotton balls.			
12. Grasps the penis gently with one hand; with the other hand, cleanses the meatus in a circular motion from the meatus outward; cleanses for a few inches down the shaft of the penis.			
13. Cleanses around the meatus at least twice, using each area of the towelette or each cotton ball only once.			
For all Patients			
NOTE: *Some lab manuals recommend rinsing the antiseptic solution from the meatus to prevent contamination of the specimen with antiseptic.*			
14. Removes gloves; washes hands; dons a second pair of clean procedure gloves.			
15. For the patient using a bedpan, raises the head of the bed to a semi-Fowler's position.			

PROCEDURE STEPS	Yes	No	COMMENTS
16. Opens the sterile specimen container; does not touch the inside of the lid or the container.			

17. Holding the container near the meatus, instructs the patient to begin voiding.
    a. For female patient: Holds the labia apart during this step (or teaches self-care patients to do so).
    b. For the male patient unable to assist, holds the penis.			

18. Allows a small stream of urine to pass, then places the specimen container into the stream.			
19. Does not let the end of the male patient's penis touch the inside of the container; does not touch the female perineum with the container.			
20. Collects approximately 30–60 mL of urine.			
21. Removes container from the stream and allows the patient to finish emptying the bladder.			
22. For the male patient who is uncircumcised, replaces the foreskin over the glans when the procedure is finished.			
23. Carefully replaces the container lid, touching only the outside of the cap and container.			
24. Cleanses the outside of the container of urine, if necessary.			
25. Labels the container with the correct patient information (in many institutions these are preprinted or bar-coded).			
26. Places the container in a facility specific carrier (usually a plastic bag) for transport to the lab.			
27. Removes gloves and washes hands. If the specimen has been obtained from a patient on a bedpan, leaves gloves on until the bedpan has been removed, emptied, and stored properly.			
28. Assists patient back to bed or removes bedpan.			
29. Transports the specimen to the lab in a timely manner.			

Recommendation: Pass _____ Needs more practice _____

Student: _____ Date: _____

Instructor: _____ Date: _____

Check (✓) Yes or No

PROCEDURE STEPS	Yes	No	COMMENTS
1. Uses sterile irrigation solution, warmed to room temperature.			
2. Never disconnects the drainage tubing from the catheter.			
3. If not already present, inserts a 3-way (triple lumen) indwelling catheter.			
4. Prepares the irrigation fluid and tubing:			
a. Closes the clamp on the connecting tubing.			
b. Spikes the tubing into the appropriate portal on the irrigation solution container, using aseptic technique.			
c. Inverts the container and hangs it on the IV pole.			
d. Removes protective cap from the distal end of the connecting tubing; holds end of tubing over a sink and opens the roller clamp slowly, allowing solution to completely fill the tubing. Recaps the tubing.			
5. Dons clean procedure gloves.			
6. Drapes patient so that only the connection port on the indwelling catheter is visible.			
7. Places a sterile barrier under the irrigation port on a 3-way catheter.			
8. Removes any plug from the port. Connects end of irrigation tubing to the side port of the catheter, using aseptic technique. Pinches or clamps tubing to prevent leakage of urine.			
9. Before beginning flow of irrigation solution, empties urine from the bedside drainage bag and documents amount.			
10. Removes gloves; washes hands.			
11. Covers the patient and makes him comfortable.			
12. Opens the roller clamp on the tubing and regulates the flow of the irrigation solution to meet the desired outcome for the irrigation (e.g., the goal of continuous bladder irrigation for patients who have had a transurethral resection of the prostate is to keep the urine light pink to clear).			

PROCEDURE STEPS	Yes	No	COMMENTS
13. Monitors flow rate for 1 to 2 minutes to ensure accuracy.			

Recommendation: Pass _____ Needs more practice _____

Student: _____   Date: _____

Instructor: _____   Date: _____

Check (✓) Yes or No

PROCEDURE STEPS	Yes	No	COMMENTS
1. Takes an extra pair of sterile gloves and an extra sterile catheter into the room.			
2. Provides good lighting; takes a procedure lamp to the bedside if necessary.			
3. Works on the right side of the bed if right-handed; the left side, if left-handed.			
4. Assists to dorsal recumbent position (knees flexed, feet flat on the bed). Instructs patient to relax her thighs and let them rotate externally (if patient is able to cooperate). Alternatively, uses Sims' position (side-lying with upper leg flexed at hip.			
5. If patient is confused, unable to follow directions, or unable to hold her legs in correct position, obtains help.			
6. Drapes patient. If dorsal recumbent position is used, folds blanket in a diamond shape, wraps corners around legs, anchors under feet, and folds upper corner down over perineum. If in Sims' position, drapes so that rectal area is covered.			
7. Dons clean procedure gloves and washes the perineal area with soap and water; dries perineal area.			
8. While washing perineum, locates the urinary meatus (for women).			
9. Removes and discards gloves.			
10. Washes hands.			
11. Organizes the work area:			
a. Bedside or over-bed table within nurse's reach.			
b. Opens sterile catheter kit and places on bedside table without contaminating the inside of the wrap.			
c. Positions a plastic bag or other trash receptacle so that nurse does not have to reach across the sterile field (e.g., near the patient's feet); or places a trash can on the floor beside the bed.			
d. Positions the procedure light or has assistant hold a flashlight.			
12. Lifts corner of privacy drape (e.g., bath blanket) to expose the perineum.			

PROCEDURE STEPS	Yes	No	COMMENTS
13. Applies sterile drape(s) and underpad. *Variation:* Waterproof underpad packed as top item in the kit.			
e. Removes the underpad from the kit before donning sterile gloves. Does not touch other kit items with bare hands. Allows drape to fall open as it is removed from the kit.			
f. Touching only the corners and shiny side, places the drape flat on the bed, shiny side down, and tucks the top edge under the patient's buttocks.			
g. Lifts corner of privacy drape (e.g., bath blanket) to expose perineum.			
h. Dons sterile gloves (from kit). (Touching only the glove package, removes it from sterile kit before donning gloves).			
i. Picks up fenestrated drape; allows it to unfold without touching other objects; places over perineum with the hole over the labia.			
Variation: Sterile gloves packed as top item in the kit. Uses the following steps instead of Steps 12 a–i:			
j. Removes gloves from package, being careful not to touch anything else in the package with bare hand. Dons gloves.			
k. Grasps the edges of the sterile underpad and folds the entire edge down 2.5 to 5 cm (1 to 2 inches) and toward self, forming a cuff to protect the sterile gloved hands.			
l. Asks patient to raise her hips slightly if she is able.			
m. Slides the drape under patient's buttocks without contaminating the gloves.			
n. Places fenestrated drape: Picks it up, allowing it to unfold without touching any other objects. Creates "cuff" to protect gloves, as in step 12(k).			
o. Places fenestrated drape so that hole is over labia.			
14. Organizes kit supplies on the sterile field and prepares the supplies in the kit, maintaining sterility.			
a. Opens the antiseptic packet; pours solution over the cotton balls. (Some kits contain sterile antiseptic swabs; if so, opens the "stick" end of the packet.)			
b. Lays forceps near cotton balls.			
c. Opens specimen container if a specimen is to be collected.			

PROCEDURE STEPS	Yes	No	COMMENTS
d. Removes any unneeded supplies (e.g., specimen container) from the field.			
e. Opens the packet of sterile lubricant and squeezes it into the kit tray.			
f. Lubricates the first 1 to 2 inches of the catheter by rolling it in the lubricant.			
15. Touching only the kit or the inside of the wrapping, places the sterile catheter kit down onto the sterile field between the patient's legs.			
16. Cleanses the urinary meatus. a. Places nondominant hand above the labia and with the thumb and forefinger spreads the patient's labia, pulls up (or anteriorly) at the same time, to expose the urinary meatus. b. Holds this position throughout the procedure—firm pressure is necessary. c. If the labia slip back over the urinary meatus, considers it contaminated and repeats cleansing procedure.			
d. Using forceps, with dominant hand, picks up a wet cotton ball and cleanses perineal area, taking care not to contaminate the sterile glove.			
e. Uses one stroke for each area.			
f. Wipes from front to back.			
g. Uses a new cotton ball for each area.			
h. Cleanses in this order: outside far labium majus, outside near labium majus, inside far labium, inside near labium, and directly down the center over the urinary meatus. (Some kits have only 3 cotton balls, so the order would be inside far labium, inside near labium, and directly down the center; the outside labia majora would have already been cleansed with soap and water.)			
17. Discards used cotton balls as they are used; does not move them across the open, sterile kit and field.			
18. Maintaining sterile technique, places the urine receptacle close enough to the urinary meatus for the end of the catheter to rest inside the container as the urine drains (4 inches or 10 cm from the meatus).			
19. Asks the woman to bear down as though she is trying to void; slowly inserts the end of the catheter into the meatus. Has the patient take slow deep breaths until the			

PROCEDURE STEPS	Yes	No	COMMENTS
initial discomfort has passed.			
20. Continues gentle insertion of catheter until urine flows. This is about 2 to 3 inches (5 to 7.5 cm) in a woman. Then inserts the catheter another 1 to 2 inches (2.5 to 5 cm).			
21. If resistance is felt, twists the catheter slightly or applies gentle pressure; does not force the catheter.			
22. If the catheter touches the labia or nonsterile linens, or is inadvertently inserted in the vagina, considers it contaminated and inserts a new, sterile catheter.			
23. If catheter is inadvertently inserted into the vagina, leaves the contaminated catheter in the vagina while inserting the new one into the meatus.			
24. Continues to hold the catheter securely with the nondominant hand while urine drains from the bladder.			
25. If a urine specimen is to be collected, uses dominant hand to place the specimen container into the flow of urine; caps container using sterile technique.			
26. When the flow of urine has ceased and the bladder has been emptied, pinches the catheter and slowly withdraws it from the meatus.			
27. Discards catheter, observing universal precautions.			
28. Removes the urine-filled receptacle and sets aside to be emptied when the procedure is finished.			
29. Cleanses patient's perineal area as needed, and dries.			
30. Removes gloves; washes hands.			
31. Returns patient to a position of comfort.			
32. Discards supplies in appropriate receptacle.			

Recommendation: Pass _____ Needs more practice _____

Student: _____   Date: _____

Instructor: _____   Date: _____

PROCEDURE CHECKLIST
Chapter 27: Inserting a Straight Urinary Catheter (Male)

Check (✓) Yes or No

PROCEDURE STEPS	Yes	No	COMMENTS
1. Takes an extra pair of sterile gloves and an extra sterile catheter into the room.			
2. Selects a catheter kit that contains lubricant in a prefilled syringe.			
3. Provides good lighting; takes a procedure lamp to the bedside if necessary.			
4. Works on the right side of the bed if right-handed; the left side, if left-handed.			
5. Places patient supine, legs straight and slightly apart.			
6. If patient is confused or unable to follow directions, obtains help.			
7. Drapes patient. Covers upper body with blanket; folds linens down to expose the penis.			
8. Dons clean procedure gloves and washes the penis and perineal area with soap and water; dries gently.			
9. If using 2% Xylocaine gel for the procedure, uses a syringe to insert it into the urethra.			
10. Removes and discards gloves.			
11. Washes hands.			
12. Organizes the work area: a. Bedside or over-bed table within nurse's reach.			
b. Opens sterile catheter kit and places on bedside table without contaminating the inside of the wrap.			
c. Positions a plastic bag or other trash receptacle so that nurse does not have to reach across the sterile field (e.g., near the patient's feet); or places a trash can on the floor beside the bed.			
13. Applies sterile drape(s) and underpad. *Variation:* Waterproof underpad packed as top item in the kit.			
a. Removes the waterproof underpad from the kit before donning sterile gloves. Does not touch other kit items with bare hands. Allows drape to fall open as it is removed from the kit.			

PROCEDURE STEPS	Yes	No	COMMENTS
b. Allows drape to fall open as it is removed from the kit. Touching only the corners and shiny side, places the drape shiny side down across top of patient's thighs.		.	
c. Dons sterile gloves (from kit). (Touching only the glove package, removes it from the sterile kit before donning the gloves.)			
d. Picks up fenestrated drape; allows it to unfold without touching other objects; places hole over the penis.			
Variation: Sterile gloves packed as top item in the kit. Uses the following steps instead of Steps 12 a-d:			
e. Removes gloves from package, being careful not to touch anything else in the package with bare hand. Dons gloves.			
f. Grasps the edges of the sterile underpad and places it shiny side down across the top of the patient's thighs.			
g. Places fenestrated drape: Picks it up, allowing it to unfold without touching any other objects. Keeps gloves sterile.			
h. Places fenestrated drape so that hole is over the penis.			
14. Organizes kit supplies on the sterile field and prepares the supplies in the kit, maintaining sterility.			
a. Opens the antiseptic packet; pours solution over the cotton balls. (Some kits contain sterile antiseptic swabs; if so, opens the "stick" end of the packet.)			
b. Lays forceps near cotton balls (omit step if kit includes swabs).			
c. Opens specimen container if a specimen is to be collected.			
d. Removes any unneeded supplies (e.g., specimen container) from the field.			
e. Expresses a small amount of sterile lubricant into the kit tray; lubricates the first 1 to 2 inches of the catheter by rolling it in the lubricant. Does not lubricate catheter if Xylocaine gel has already been inserted into the urethra (Step 9).			
15. With nondominant hand, reaches through the opening in the fenestrated drape and grasps the penis, taking care not to contaminate the surrounding drape. If penis is uncircumcised, retracts foreskin with nondominant hand to expose the meatus.			

PROCEDURE STEPS	Yes	No	COMMENTS
16. If the foreskin accidentally falls back over the meatus, or if the nurse drops the penis during cleansing, repeats the procedure.			
17. Continuing to hold the penis with the nondominant hand, holds forceps in dominant hand and picks up a cotton ball.			
18. Beginning at the meatus, cleanses the glans in a circular motion in ever-widening circles and partially down the shaft of the penis.			
19. Repeats with at least one more cotton ball.			
20. Discards cotton balls as they are used; does not move them across the open, sterile kit and field.			
21. Maintaining sterile technique, places the plastic urine receptacle close enough to the urinary meatus for the end of the catheter to rest inside the container as the urine drains (e.g., places container between patient's thighs)			
22. Using the nondominant hand, holds the penis gently but firmly at a 90° angle to the body, exerting gentle traction.			
23. Gently inserts the tip of the prefilled syringe into the urethra and instill the lubricant. (If the kit contains only a single packet of lubricant and if no other kits are available, lubricates 5 to 7 inches (12.5 to 17.7 cm) of the catheter. This is not the technique of choice, however.)			
24. With the dominant hand, holds the catheter 3 inches (7.5 cm) from the proximal end, with remainder coiled in the palm of the hand; or otherwise ensures that the distal end of the catheter is in the plastic container.			
25. Asks the patient to bear down as though trying to void; slowly inserts the end of the catheter into the meatus. Has the patient take slow deep breaths until the initial discomfort has passed.			
26. Continues gentle insertion of catheter until urine flows. This is about 7 to 9 inches (17 to 22.5 cm) in a man. Then inserts the catheter another 1 to 2 inches (2.5 to 5 cm).			
27. If resistance is felt, withdraws the catheter; does not force the catheter.			
28. Continues to hold the penis and catheter securely in hand while the urine drains from the bladder.			

PROCEDURE STEPS	Yes	No	COMMENTS
29. If a urine specimen is to be collected, uses dominant hand to place the specimen container into the flow of urine; caps container using sterile technique.			
30. When the flow of urine has ceased and the bladder has been emptied, pinches the catheter and slowly withdraws it from the meatus.			
31. Discards catheter.			
32. Removes the urine-filled receptacle and sets aside to be emptied when the procedure is finished.			
33. Cleanses and dries patient's penis and perineal area as needed; replaces foreskin over end of penis.			
34. Removes gloves; washes hands.			
35. Returns patient to a position of comfort.			
36. Discards supplies in appropriate receptacle.			

Recommendation: Pass _____ Needs more practice _____

Student: _____   Date: _____

Instructor: _____   Date: _____

PROCEDURE CHECKLIST
Chapter 27: Inserting an Indwelling Urinary Catheter (Female)

Check (✓) Yes or No

PROCEDURE STEPS	Yes	No	COMMENTS
1. Takes an extra pair of sterile gloves and an extra sterile catheter into the room.			
2. Provides good lighting; takes a procedure lamp to the bedside if necessary.			
3. Works on the right side of the bed if right-handed; the left side, if left-handed.			
4. Assists to dorsal recumbent position (knees flexed, feet flat on the bed). Instructs patient to relax her thighs and let them rotate externally (if patient is able to cooperate). Alternatively, uses Sims' position (side-lying with upper leg flexed at hip.			
5. If patient is confused, unable to follow directions, or unable to hold her legs in correct position, obtains help.			
6. Drapes patient. If dorsal recumbent position is used, folds blanket in a diamond shape, wraps corners around legs, anchors under feet, and folds upper corner down over perineum. If in Sims' position, drapes so that rectal area is covered.			
7. Dons clean procedure gloves and washes the perineal area with soap and water; dries perineal area.			
8. While washing perineum, locates the urinary meatus.			
9. Removes and discards gloves.			
10. Washes hands.			
11. Organizes the work area:			
a. Bedside or over-bed table within nurse's reach.			
b. Opens sterile catheter kit and places on bedside table without contaminating the inside of the wrap.			
c. Positions a plastic bag or other trash receptacle so that nurse does not have to reach across the sterile field (e.g., near the patient's feet); or places a trash can on the floor beside the bed.			
d. Positions the procedure light or has assistant hold a flashlight.			
e. Lifts corner of privacy drape (e.g., bath blanket) to expose perineum.			
12. Applies sterile drape(s) and underpad.			

PROCEDURE STEPS	Yes	No	COMMENTS
Variation: Waterproof underpad packed as top item in the kit.			
f. Removes the underpad from the kit before donning sterile gloves. Does not touch other kit items with bare hands. Allows drape to fall open as it is removed from the kit.			
g. Touching only the corners and shiny side, places the drape flat on the bed, shiny side down, and tucks the top edge under the patient's buttocks.			
h. Lifts corner of privacy drape (e.g., bath blanket) to expose perineum.			
i. Dons sterile gloves (from kit). (Touching only the glove package, removes it from sterile kit before donning gloves).			
j. Picks up fenestrated drape; allows it to unfold without touching other objects; places over perineum with the hole over the labia.			
Variation: Sterile gloves packed as top item in the kit.			
Uses the following steps instead of Steps 12 a-j: k. Removes gloves from package, being careful not to touch anything else in the package with bare hand. Dons gloves. l. Grasps the edges of the sterile underpad and folds the entire edge down 2.5 to 5 cm (1 to 2 inches) and toward self, forming a cuff to protect the sterile gloved hands. m. Asks patient to raise her hips slightly if she is able. n. Slides the drape under patient's buttocks without contaminating the gloves. o. Places fenestrated drape: Picks it up, allowing it to unfold without touching any other objects. Creates "cuff" to protect gloves, as in step 12-l. p. Places fenestrated drape so that hole is over labia.			
13. Organizes kit supplies on the sterile field and prepares the supplies in the kit, maintaining sterility.			
a. Opens the antiseptic packet; pours solution over the cotton balls. (Some kits contain sterile antiseptic swabs; if so, opens the "stick" end of the packet.)			
b. Lays forceps near cotton balls (omits step if using swabs).			
c. Opens specimen container if a specimen is to be collected.			
d. Removes any unneeded supplies (e.g., specimen container) from the field.			
e. Removes plastic covering from catheter.			

PROCEDURE STEPS	Yes	No	COMMENTS
f. Opens package and expresses sterile lubricant into the kit tray; lubricates the first 1 to 2 inches (2.5 to 5 cm) of the catheter by rolling it in the lubricant.			
g. Removes plastic cover from catheter. Attaches the saline-filled syringe to the side port of the catheter and inflates the balloon.			
h. Deflates balloon and returns catheter to the kit, leaving the syringe connected to the port.			
14. Touching only the sterile box or inside of the wrapping, places the sterile catheter kit (tray and box) down onto the sterile field between the patient's legs.			
15. If the drainage bag is preconnected to the catheter itself, leaves the bag on or near the sterile field until after the catheter is inserted.			
16. Cleanses the urinary meatus.			
a. Places nondominant hand above the labia and with the thumb and forefinger spreads the patient's labia, pulls up (or anteriorly) at the same time, to expose the urinary meatus.			
b. Holds this position throughout the procedure—firm pressure is necessary.			
c. If the labia slip back over the urinary meatus, considers it contaminated and repeats cleansing procedure.			
d. With dominant hand, picks up a wet cotton ball (or swab), using forceps, and cleanses perineal area, taking care not to contaminate the sterile glove.			
e. Uses one stroke for each area.			
f. Wipes from front to back..			
g. Uses a new cotton ball for each area.			
h. Cleanses in this order: outside far labium majus, outside near labium majus, inside far labium, inside near labium, and directly down the center over the urinary meatus. If there are only 3 cotton balls in the kit, labia majora should be washed with soap and water initially; and in this step, cleanses only the inside far labium majus, inside near labium, and down center directly over the meatus.			
17. Discards used cotton balls or swabs as they are used; does not move them across the open, sterile kit and field.			
18. With the dominant hand, holds the catheter approximately 3 inches (7.5 cm) from the proximal end; coils remainder of catheter in palm of hand or otherwise protects it from contamination.			

PROCEDURE STEPS	Yes	No	COMMENTS
19. Asks the woman to bear down as though she is trying to void; slowly inserts the end of the catheter into the meatus. Has the patient take slow deep breaths until the initial discomfort has passed.			
20. Continues gentle insertion of catheter until urine flows. This is about 2 to 3 inches (5 to 7.5 cm) in a woman. Then inserts the catheter another 1 to 2 inches (2.5 to 5 cm).			
21. If resistance is felt, twists the catheter slightly or applies gentle pressure; does not force the catheter.			
22. If the catheter touches the labia or nonsterile linens, or is inadvertently inserted in the vagina, considers it contaminated and inserts a new, sterile catheter.			
23. If catheter is inadvertently inserted into the vagina, leaves the contaminated catheter in the vagina while inserting the new one into the meatus.			
24. Continues to hold the catheter securely with the dominant hand; after urine flows, stabilizes the catheter's position in the urethra and uses the nondominant hand to pick up the saline-filled syringe and inflate the catheter balloon.			
25. If the patient complains of severe pain upon inflation of the balloon, the catheter is probably in the urethra. Allows the water to drain out of the balloon and repositions the catheter by advancing it 1 inch (2.5 cm).			
26. Connects the drainage bag to the end of the catheter if it is not already preconnected. Hangs the drainage bag on the side of the bed, below the level of the bladder.			
27. Using a tape or a catheter strap, secures the catheter to the thigh.			
28. Cleanses patients perineal area as needed, and dries.			
29. Removes gloves; washes hands.			
30. Returns patient to a position of comfort.			
31. Discards supplies in appropriate receptacle.			

Recommendation: Pass _____ Needs more practice _____

Student: _____   Date: _____

Instructor: _____   Date: _____

PROCEDURE CHECKLIST
Chapter 27: Inserting an Indwelling Urinary Catheter (Male)

Check (✓) Yes or No

PROCEDURE STEPS	Yes	No	COMMENTS
1. Takes an extra pair of sterile gloves and an extra sterile catheter into the room.			
2. Selects a catheter kit that contains lubricant in a prefilled syringe.			
3. Provides good lighting; takes a procedure lamp to the bedside if necessary.			
4. Works on the right side of the bed if right-handed; the left side, if left-handed.			
5. Places patient supine, legs straight and slightly apart.			
6. If patient is confused or unable to follow directions, obtains help.			
7. Drapes patient. Covers upper body with blanket; folds linens down to expose the penis.			
8. Dons clean procedure gloves and washes the penis and perineal area with soap and water; dries gently.			
9. If using 2% Xylocaine gel for the procedure, uses a syringe and inserts it into the urethra.			
10. Removes and discards gloves.			
11. Washes hands.			
12. Organizes the work area:			
a. Bedside or over-bed table within nurse's reach.			
b. Opens sterile catheter kit and places on bedside table, without contaminating the inside of the wrap.			
c. Positions a plastic bag or other trash receptacle so that nurse does not have to reach across the sterile field (e.g., near the patient's feet); or places a trash can on the floor beside the bed.			
13. Applies sterile drape(s) and underpad. *Variation:* Waterproof underpad packed as top item in the kit.			
a. Removes the waterproof underpad from the kit before donning sterile gloves. Does not touch other kit items with bare hands. Allows drape to fall open as it is removed from the kit.			

PROCEDURE STEPS	Yes	No	COMMENTS
b. Allows drape to fall open as it is removed from the kit. Touching only the corners and shiny side, places the drape shiny side down across top of patient's thighs.			
c. Dons sterile gloves (from kit). (Touching only the glove package, removes it from the sterile kit before donning the gloves.)			
d. Picks up fenestrated drape; allows it to unfold without touching other objects; places hole over the penis.			
Variation: Sterile gloves packed as top item in the kit.			
Uses the following steps instead of Steps 12 a–d: e. Removes gloves from package, being careful not to touch anything else in the package with bare hand. Dons gloves. f. Grasps the edges of the sterile underpad and places it shiny side down across the top of the patient's thighs. g. Places fenestrated drape: Picks it up, allowing it to unfold without touching any other objects. Keeps gloves sterile. h. Places fenestrated drape so that hole is over the penis.			
14. Organizes kit supplies on the sterile field and prepares the supplies in the kit, maintaining sterility.			
a. Opens the antiseptic packet; pours solution over the cotton balls. (Some kits contain sterile antiseptic swabs; if so, opens the "stick" end of the packet.)			
b. Lays forceps near cotton balls (omit step if using swabs).			
c. Opens specimen container if a specimen is to be collected.			
d. Removes any unneeded supplies (e.g., specimen container) from the field.			
e. Expresses a small amount of sterile lubricant into the kit tray; lubricates the first 1 to 2 inches of the catheter by rolling it in the lubricant. Does not lubricate catheter if Xylocaine gel has already been inserted into the urethra in step 9.			
f. Attaches the saline-filled syringe to the side port of the catheter and checks balloon by inflating; deflates balloon and returns it and the catheter to the kit. Leaves syringe attached to catheter.			

PROCEDURE STEPS	Yes	No	COMMENTS
15. Touching only the kit or inside of the wrapping, places the sterile catheter kit down onto the sterile field between or on top of the patient's thighs.			
16. If the drainage bag is preconnected to the catheter, leaves the bag on the sterile field until after the catheter is inserted.			
17. With nondominant hand, reaches through the opening in the fenestrated drape and grasps the penis, taking care not to contaminate the surrounding drape. If penis is uncircumcised, retracts foreskin to expose the meatus.			
18. If the foreskin accidentally falls back over the meatus, or if the nurse drops the penis during cleansing, repeats the procedure.			
19. Continuing to hold the penis with the nondominant hand, holds forceps in dominant hand and picks up a cotton ball.			
20. Beginning at the meatus, cleanses the glans in a circular motion in ever-widening circles and partially down the shaft of the penis.			
21. Repeats with at least one more cotton ball.			
22. Discards cotton balls or swabs as they are used; does not move them across the open, sterile kit and field.			
23. Using the nondominant hand, holds the penis gently but firmly at a 90° angle to the body, exerting gentle traction.			
24. Gently inserts the tip of the prefilled syringe into the urethra and instill the lubricant. (If the kit contains only a single packet of lubricant and if no other kits are available, then lubricates 5 to 7 inches (12.5 to 17.7 cm) of the catheter. This is not the technique of choice, however.)			
25. With the dominant hand, holds the catheter 3 inches (7.5 cm) from the proximal end, with remainder of the catheter coiled in palm of hand.			
26. Asks the patient to bear down as though trying to void; slowly inserts the end of the catheter into the meatus. Has the patient take slow deep breaths until the initial discomfort has passed.			
27. Continues gentle insertion of catheter until urine flows. This is about 7 to 9 inches (17 to 22.5 cm) in a man. Then inserts the catheter another 1 to 2 inches (2.5 to 5 cm).			

PROCEDURE STEPS	Yes	No	COMMENTS
28. If resistance is felt, withdraws the catheter; does not force the catheter.			
29. After urine flows, stabilizes the catheter's position in the urethra with nondominant hand; uses dominant hand to pick up saline-filled syringe and inflate catheter balloon.			
30. If patient complains of severe pain upon inflation of the balloon, the balloon is probably in the urethra. Allows the water to drain out of the balloon, and advances the catheter 1 inch (2.5) farther into the bladder.			
31. If it is not preconnected, connects the drainage bag to the end of the catheter.			
32. Hangs the drainage bag on the side of the bed below the level of the bladder.			
33. Using tape or a catheter strap, secures the catheter to the thigh or the abdomen.			
34. Cleanses patient's penis and perineal area as needed, and dries. Ensures that foreskin is no longer retracted.			
35. Removes gloves; washes hands.			
36. Returns patient to a position of comfort.			
37. Discards supplies in appropriate receptacle.			

Recommendation: Pass _____ Needs more practice _____

Student: _____   Date: _____

Instructor: _____   Date: _____

PROCEDURE CHECKLIST
Chapter 27: Intermittent Bladder or Catheter Irrigation

Check (✓) Yes or No

PROCEDURE STEPS	Yes	No	COMMENTS
1. Uses sterile irrigation solution, warmed to room temperature.			
2. Never disconnects the drainage tubing from the catheter.			
3. If not already present, inserts a 3-way (triple lumen) indwelling catheter.			
Intermittent Irrigation, Three-way (Triple Lumen) Indwelling catheter			
4. Prepares the irrigation fluid and tubing: a. Closes the clamp on the connecting tubing.			
b. Spikes the tubing into the appropriate portal on the irrigation solution container, using aseptic technique.			
c. Inverts the container and hangs it on the IV pole.			
d. Removes protective cap from the distal end of the connecting tubing; holds end of tubing over a sink and opens the roller clamp slowly, allowing solution to completely fill the tubing. Recaps the tubing.			
5. Dons clean procedure gloves.			
6. Drapes patient so that only the connection port on the indwelling catheter is visible.			
7. Prior to beginning the flow of irrigation solution, empties any urine that may be in the bedside drainage bag and documents amount.			
8. Determines whether the irrigant is to remain in the bladder for any length of time. If irrigant is to remain in the bladder for a certain time period, clamps the drainage tubing for that time.			
9. Slowly opens roller clamp on the irrigation tubing.			
10. Instills or irrigates with the prescribed amount of irrigant.			
11. When the correct amount of irrigant has been used and/or the goals of the irrigation have been met, closes the roller clamp on the irrigation tubing, leaving the tubing connected to the catheter for use during the next irrigation.			

PROCEDURE STEPS	Yes	No	COMMENTS
12. Removes gloves; washes hands.			
13. Makes patient comfortable.			
Intermittent Irrigation, Two-Way Indwelling Catheter			
14. Dons clean procedure gloves; empties any urine currently in the bedside drainage bag.			
15. Drapes patient so that only the specimen removal port on the drainage tubing is exposed.			
16. Places a waterproof drape beneath the exposed port.			
17. Opens the sterile irrigation supplies. Pours approximately 100 mL of the irrigating solution into the sterile container, using aseptic technique.			
18. Swabs specimen removal port with antiseptic swab.			
19. Draws irrigation solution into the syringe. (For catheter irrigation, use a total of 30–40 mL; for bladder irrigation the amount is usually 100–200 mL.)			
20. Inserts the needle into the specimen port. Points the needle toward the bladder.			
21. Holds the specimen port with the fingers; does not lay the tubing/port in the palm of the hand when accessing the port.			
22. Clamps drainage tubing distal to the specimen port.			
23. Injects the solution, holding the specimen port slightly above the level of the bladder.			
24. If meets resistance, has patient turn slightly and attempts a second time. If resistance continues, stops the procedure and notifies the physician.			
25. When the irrigant has been injected, withdraws the needle. Refills the syringe if necessary.			
26. Does NOT recap the needle. If necessary to repeat the irrigation, rests the needle end of the syringe in the irrigation solution container.			
27. Unclamps the drainage tubing and allows the irrigant and urine to flow into the bedside drainage bag by gravity. (If the solution is to remain in the bladder for a prescribed time, leaves the tubing clamped for that time period.)			

PROCEDURE STEPS	Yes	No	COMMENTS
28. Repeats the procedure as necessary until the prescribed amount has been instilled, or until the goal of the irrigation is met. (e.g. removal of clots, mucus, urine flowing freely, etc.)			
29. Removes gloves, washes hands.			
30. Returns patient to a position of comfort.			

Recommendation: Pass _____ Needs more practice _____

Student: _____   Date: _____

Instructor: _____   Date: _____

PROCEDURE CHECKLIST
Chapter 28: Administering a Cleansing Enema

Check (✓) Yes or No

PROCEDURE STEPS	Yes	No	COMMENTS
1. Determines patient's ability to retain the enema solution.			
2. Places a bedpan or bedside commode nearby for the patient with limited mobility.			
3. Warms the solution to 105°–110°F —not in a microwave. Checks temperature with bath thermometer.			
4. Opens the enema kit or obtains supplies.			
5. Attaches tubing to the enema bucket if a bucket is being used (the 1-liter enema bag comes with preconnected tubing).			
6. Closes the clamp on the tubing and fills the container with 500–1100 mL of warm solution (40–150 mL for infants; 250–350 mL for toddlers; 300–500 mL for school-age children).			
7. Checks water with a bath thermometer. Temperature should be 105–110 degrees F (lukewarm).			
8. Adds Castile soap or soap solution used by the facility, if a soapsuds enema was ordered.			
9. Hangs the container on the IV pole.			
10. Holding the end of the tubing over a sink or waste can, opens the clamp and slowly allows the tubing to prime (fill) with solution. Reclamps when filled.			
11. Has the patient turn or assists to turn to a left side-lying position with the right knee flexed. (Elevates head of the bed very slightly for patients who have shortness of breath.)			
12. Drapes patient with bath blanket, leaving only the buttocks and rectum exposed.			
13. Dons clean procedure gloves.			
14. Places a waterproof pad under the patient's buttocks/hips.			
15. Places the bedpan flat on the bed directly beneath the rectum, up against the patient's buttocks; or places the bedside commode near the bed.			
16. Generously lubricates the tip of the enema tubing.			
17. If necessary, lifts the superior buttock to expose the anus.			
18. Slowly and gently inserts tip of the tubing approximately 3 to 4 inches (7 to 10 cm) into the rectum; asks patient to take slow, deep breaths during this step.			

PROCEDURE STEPS	Yes	No	COMMENTS
19. If tube does not pass with ease, does not force; allows a small amount of fluid to infuse and then tries again.			
20. Removes the container from the IV pole and holds it at the level of the patient's hips. Begins instilling the solution.			
21. Slowly raises the level of the container so that it is 12 to 18 inches (30–45 cm) above the level of the hips. Adjusts the IV pole and rehangs the container.			
22. Continues a slow, steady instillation of the enema solution.			
23. Continuously monitors the patient for pain or discomfort. If pain occurs or resistance is met at any time during procedure, stops and consults with primary care provider.			
24. Assesses ability to retain the solution. If the patient has difficulty with retention, lowers the level of the container, stops the flow for 15–30 seconds, and then resumes the procedure.			
25. When the correct amount of solution has been instilled, clamps the tubing and slowly removes the tubing from the rectum.			
26. If there is stool on the tubing, wraps the end of the tubing in a washcloth or toilet tissue until it can be rinsed or disposed of.			
27. Cleanses the patient's rectal area.			
28. Re-covers the patient.			
29. Instructs patient to hold the enema solution for 5 to 10 minutes.			
30. Places call light within reach.			
31. Disposes of enema supplies or, if reusable, cleans and stores in an appropriate location in the patient's room.			
32. Removes gloves; washes hands.			
33. Depending on the patient's mobility status, assists onto the bedpan, to the bedside commode, or to the toilet when she feels compelled to defecate.			
34. After the patient has defecated, inspects the stool for color, consistency, and quantity.			

Recommendation: Pass _____ Needs more practice _____

Student: _____   Date: _____

Instructor: _____   Date: _____

PROCEDURE CHECKLIST
Chapter 28: Administering a Prepackaged Enema

Check (✓) Yes or No

PROCEDURE STEPS	Yes	No	COMMENTS
1. Determines patient's ability to retain the enema solution.			
2. Places a bedpan or bedside commode nearby for the patient with limited mobility.			
3. Warms the solution—not in a microwave.			
4. Has the patient turn or assists to turn to a left side-lying position with the right knee flexed. (Elevates head of the bed very slightly for patients who have shortness of breath.)			
5. Drapes patient with bath blanket, leaving only the buttocks and rectum exposed.			
6. Dons clean procedure gloves.			
7. Places a waterproof pad under the patient's buttocks/hips.			
8. Opens the prepackaged enema. Removes the plastic cap from the container. The tip of the prepackaged enema container comes prelubricated. Adds extra lubricant as needed.			
9. If necessary, lifts the superior buttock to expose the anus.			
10. Slowly and gently inserts tip of the tubing approximately 3 to 4 inches (7 to 10 cm) into the rectum; asks patient to take slow, deep breaths during this step.			
11. If tube does not insert with ease, does not force; removes, relubricates, and retries.			
12. Tilts container slightly and slowly rolls and squeezes the container until all of the solution is instilled.			
13. Withdraws container tip from the rectum; wipes the area with a washcloth or toilet tissue.			
14. Cleans the patient's rectal area, re-covers the patient and instructs to hold the enema solution for approximately 5–10 minutes.			
15. Removes gloves; washes hands.			
16. Places call light within reach.			
17. Disposes of empty container.			
18. Depending on the patient's mobility status, assists onto the bedpan, to the bedside commode, or to the toilet when she feels compelled to defecate.			

PROCEDURE STEPS	Yes	No	COMMENTS

Recommendation: Pass _____ Needs more practice _____

Student: _____ Date: _____

Instructor: _____ Date: _____

PROCEDURE CHECKLIST
Chapter 28: Changing an Ostomy Appliance

Check (✓) Yes or No

PROCEDURE STEPS	Yes	No	COMMENTS
1. Washes hands and dons clean procedure gloves.			
2. Folds down the linens to expose the ostomy site; places a clean towel across the patient's abdomen under the existing pouch.			
3. Positions the patient so that no skin folds occur along the line of the stoma.			
4. If the pouch is drainable, opens it by removing the clamp and unrolling it at the bottom.			
5. Empties the existing ostomy pouch into a bedpan.			
6. Saves the clamp for re-use (note that some pouches cannot be drained).			
7. With one hand, gently removes the old wafer from the skin, beginning at the top and proceeding in a downward direction. At the same time, uses the other hand to hold tension on the skin in the opposite direction of the pull.			
8. If resistance is encountered and the wafer is difficult to remove, uses adhesive remover or rubbing alcohol, according to facility protocol.			
9. Places the old pouch and wafer in a plastic bag for disposal. If the pouch is nondrainable, disposes of it according to agency protocol.			
10. Inspects stoma and peristomal skin.			
11. Uses warm water and mild soap to cleanse stoma and surrounding skin.			
12. Reports excess bleeding to the physician.			
13. Allows the area to dry.			
14. Measures the size of the stoma in one of the following ways: a. Using a standard stoma measuring guide placed over the stoma. b. Re-using a previously cut template. c. Measuring the stoma from side to side (approximating the circumference).			
15. Places a clean 4×4 gauze pad over the stoma.			
16. Removes gloves and washes hands.			

PROCEDURE STEPS	Yes	No	COMMENTS
17. Traces the size of the opening obtained in Step 14 onto the paper on the back of the new wafer; cuts the opening. Wafer opening is approximately 1/16 to 1/8 inch (1.5–3 cm) larger than the circumference of the stoma.			
18. Peels the paper off the wafer. Some resources suggest first holding the wafer between the palms of the hands to warm the adhesive ring.			
19. **NOTE:** Some ostomy wafers come with an outer ring of tape attached. If so, does not remove the backing on this tape until the wafer is securely positioned (Steps 22–24).			
20. If ostomy skin care products are to be used, applies them at this time (e.g., wipes around stoma with skin-prep, applies skin barrier powder or paste, applies extra adhesive paste).			
21. Dons clean procedure gloves.			
22. Removes the gauze. Centers the wafer opening around the stoma and gently presses down.			

a. If using a one-piece pouch, makes sure the bag is pointed toward the patient's feet.
    b. If using a two-piece system, places the wafer on first. When the seal is complete, attaches the bag following manufacturer's instructions.
    c. For an open-ended pouch, folds the end of the pouch over the clamp and closes the clamp, listening for a "click" to ensure it is secure.			

23. Asks the patient to place her hand over the newly applied wafer to warm the adhesive ring, making it adhere better. Some sources also suggest taping down the edges of the wafer.			
24. Removes gloves and washes hands.			
25. Returns patient to a comfortable position.			
26. Disposes of used ostomy pouch following agency policy for biohazardous waste.			

Recommendation: Pass _____ Needs more practice _____

Student: _____   Date: _____

Instructor: _____   Date: _____

PROCEDURE CHECKLIST
Chapter 28: Irrigating a Colostomy

Check (✓) Yes or No

PROCEDURE STEPS	Yes	No	COMMENTS
1. Places IV pole near where the procedure will take place (e.g., in the bathroom, next to the bedside commode, or next to the bed).			
2. Assists the patient to the bathroom (if possible).			
3. Asks the patient if she prefers to sit directly on the toilet or on a chair in front of it.			

4. Prepares the irrigation container.
    a. For two-piece systems, connects the tubing to the container.
    b. Clamps the tubing. Fills the container with 500–1000 mL of warm tap water.			

5. Primes the tubing; unclamps the tubing to allow for filling.			
6. Hangs the solution container on the IV pole. Adjusts the IV pole to be at the height of the patient's shoulder (approximately 18 inches, or 45 cm, above the stoma).			
7. Washes hands and dons clean procedure gloves.			
8. Removes the existing colostomy appliance (if patient is wearing one) following the steps in Procedure Checklist Chapter 28: Changing an Ostomy Appliance.			
9. Inspects the stoma and surrounding skin area.			
10. Disposes of the used colostomy appliance properly. Empties contents into bedpan or toilet and discards the pouch in a moisture-proof (e.g., plastic) bag.			

11. Applies the colostomy irrigation sleeve, following manufacturer's directions.
    a. Sleeves with adhesive backing are applied following pouch application steps found in Procedure Checklist Chapter 28: Changing an Ostomy Appliance.
    b. For sleeves without an adhesive backing, places the belt around the patient's waist and attaches ends to the pouch flange on either side.
    c. For patients sitting in front of the toilet or bedside commode, places a waterproof pad under the sleeve over the patient's thighs.			

12. **Note**: For patients sitting directly on a toilet or bedside commode, the end of the sleeve should hang down past the patient's pubic area, but not down into the water. For a patient in bed, the end of the sleeve should go into the bedpan.			

PROCEDURE STEPS	Yes	No	COMMENTS
13. Generously lubricates the cone at the end of the irrigation tubing with water-soluble lubricant.			
14. Opens the top of the irrigation sleeve; inserts the cone gently into the colostomy stoma and holds it solidly in place.			
15. Opens the clamp on the tubing and slowly begins the flow of water. The fluid should flow in at a rate of about 1 liter per 5 to 10 minutes, or as the patient can tolerate.			
16. If the patient complains of discomfort, stops the flow for 15–30 seconds and has the patient take deep breaths.			
17. When the correct amount of solution has instilled, clamps the tubing and removes the cone from the stoma.			
18. Wraps the end of the cone in tissue or paper towel until it can be cleaned or disposed of properly.			
19. Closes the top of the irrigation sleeve with a clamp.			
20. Has the patient remain sitting until most of the irrigation fluid and bowel contents have evacuated. **Note**: Can also clamp the end of the sleeve and have the patient ambulate to stimulate compete evacuation of stool.			
21. When evacuation is complete, opens the top clamp, rinses and removes the irrigation sleeve. Sets it aside.			
22. Cleanses the stoma and peristomal area with a warm washcloth; allows to dry.			
23. Applies a new colostomy appliance, if patient is wearing one, following the steps in Procedure Checklist Chapter 28: Changing an Ostomy Appliance. Otherwise, covers the stoma with a small gauze bandage.			
24. Cleans the irrigation sleeve with mild soap and water. Allows it to dry.			
25. Places the irrigation supplies in the proper place (e.g., in a plastic container or plastic bag).			
26. Removes gloves and washes hands.			
27. Assists the patient back to a position of comfort.			

Recommendation: Pass _____ Needs more practice _____

Student: _____   Date: _____

Instructor: _____   Date: _____

PROCEDURE CHECKLIST
Chapter 28: Placing and Removing a Bedpan

Check (✓) Yes or No

PROCEDURE STEPS	Yes	No	COMMENTS
1. Determines whether patient needs regular bedpan or fracture pan.			
2. Obtains the necessary supplies and proceeds to the patient's room. Leaves clean washcloths, towel, and basin with warm water at the bedside for use during bedpan removal.			
3. If the bedpan is metal, places it under warm, running water for a few seconds; then dries, making sure bedpan is not too hot.			
4. Raises side rail on the opposite side of the bed, if not already up.			
5. Raises the bed to a comfortable working height.			
6. Prepares the patient by folding down the covers to a point that will allow placement of the bedpan.			
7. Dons clean procedure gloves.			
For Patients Who are Able to Move/Turn Independently in Bed			
8. Notes the presence of dressings, drains, intravenous fluids, and traction.			
9. Places patient supine; lowers the head of the bed.			
10a. Asks the patient to lift his hips. The patient may need to raise his knees to a flexed position, place his feet flat on the bed and push up. Slides a hand under the small of the patient's back, as needed, to assist the patient. 10b. Alternatively, places patient in a semi-Fowler's position; asks him to raise his hips by pushing up on raised side rails or by using an over-bed trapeze.			
11. Places the bedpan under the patient's buttocks with the wide, rounded end toward the back. When using a fracture pan, places the wide, rounded end toward the front.			
12. Does not "push" the pan under the patient's buttocks.			
13. Repositions the patient: a. Replaces the covers; raises the head of the bed to a position of comfort for the patient.			
b. Places a rolled towel, blanket, or small pillow under the sacrum (lumbar curve of the back).			

PROCEDURE STEPS	Yes	No	COMMENTS
c. Places the call light and toilet tissue within the patient's reach.			
d. Places bed back in its lowest position and raises both upper side rails.			
14. Removes gloves and washes hands.			
For patients Who Are Unable to Move/Turn Independently			
15. Asks for help from another healthcare worker, as needed.			
16. With patient supine, lowers the head of the bed.			
17. Assists patient to a side-lying position, using a turning sheet if necessary.			
18. Places the bedpan up against the patient's buttocks with the wide, rounded end toward the head. When using a fracture pan, places the wide rounded end toward the feet.			
19. Holding the bedpan in place, slowly rolls the patient back and onto the bedpan.			
20. Repositions the patient:			
a. Replaces the covers; raises the head of the bed to a position of comfort for the patient.			
b. Places a rolled towel, blanket, or small pillow under the sacrum (lumbar curve of the back).			
c. Places the call light and toilet tissue within the patient's reach.			
d. Places bed back in its lowest position and raises both upper side rails.			
21. Removes gloves and washes hands.			
Removing the Bedpan			
22. Dons clean procedure gloves.			
23. Wets the washcloth(s) with warm water and places near the work area.			
24. Lowers head of bed; raises bed to comfortable working height.			
25. Pulls covers down only as far as necessary to remove the bedpan.			
26. Offers the patient toilet paper (assists as needed).			
27. Asks the patient to raise her hips. Stabilizes and removes the bedpan. If the patient is unable to raise her hips, stabilizes the bedpan and assists her to the side-lying position.			

PROCEDURE STEPS	Yes	No	COMMENTS
28. Cleanses the buttocks with a warm, wet washcloth; dries with a towel.			
29. Replaces covers and positions patient for comfort.			
30. Offers the second warm, moistened washcloth to the patient to cleanse her hands.			
31. Empties the bedpan in the patient's toilet.			
32. Measures output if I&O is part of the treatment plan.			
33. Cleans bedpan following facility guidelines.			
34. Removes soiled gloves and washes hands.			

Recommendation: Pass _____ Needs more practice _____

Student: _____   Date: _____

Instructor: _____   Date: _____

PROCEDURE CHECKLIST
Chapter 28: Removing Stool Digitally

Check (✓) Yes or No

PROCEDURE STEPS	Yes	No	COMMENTS
1. Trims and files own fingernails if they extend over the end of the fingertips.			
2. Obtains baseline vital signs and determines whether the patient has a history of cardiac problems or other contraindications.			
3. Checks to see if an oil retention enema is ordered prior to and/or after the procedure. Administers, if so.			
4. Obtains correct lubricant (e.g., Lidocaine, if ordered).			
5. Assists patient to turn to his left side with his right knee flexed toward his head.			
6. Places a waterproof pad halfway beneath the left hip.			
7. Drapes patient to expose only the rectal area.			
8. Dons clean procedure gloves; double gloves if desired or if dictated by policy.			
9. Exposes patient's buttocks; places a clean, dry bedpan on the waterproof pad, next to the buttocks.			
10. Wets a washcloth or places toilet tissue or moist towelette nearby to cleanse rectal area upon completion of the procedure.			
11. Generously lubricates the gloved forefinger and/or middle finger of the dominant hand.			
12. Slowly slides one lubricated finger into the rectum. Observes for perianal irritation.			
13. Gently rotates the finger around the mass and/or into the mass.			
14. Begins to break the stool into smaller pieces. One method is to insert a second finger and gently "slice" apart the stool using a scissoring motion. Removes pieces of stool as they become separated, and places them in the bedpan.			
15. Instructs the patient to take slow, deep breaths during the procedure.			
16. Allowing patient to rest at intervals, continues to manipulate and remove pieces of stool.			
17. Reapplies lubricant each time fingers are reinserted.			

PROCEDURE STEPS	Yes	No	COMMENTS
18. Assesses the patient's heart rate at regular intervals. Stops the procedure if heart rate falls or rhythm changes from the initial assessment.			
19. Depending on agency policy and nursing judgment, limits session to four finger insertions and gives a suppository between subsequent sessions.			
20. When removal of stool is complete, covers bedpan and sets aside.			
21. Uses washcloth and/or toilet tissue to cleanse the rectal area.			
22. Assists patient to a position of comfort.			
23. Notes color, amount, and consistency of stool.			
24. Disposes of stool and cleans bedpan properly.			
25. Removes gloves and washes hands.			

Recommendation: Pass _____ Needs more practice _____

Student: _____   Date: _____

Instructor: _____   Date: _____

PROCEDURE CHECKLIST
Chapter 28: Testing Stool for Occult Blood

Check (✓) Yes or No

PROCEDURE STEPS	Yes	No	COMMENTS
1. Determines whether the test will be done by the nurse at the point of service or by lab personnel.			
2. Has the patient void before collecting the stool specimen.			
3. Dons procedure gloves.			
4. Places a clean, dry container for the stool specimen into the toilet or bedside commode in such a manner that the urine falls into the toilet and the fecal specimen falls into the container. Obtains a clean, dry bedpan for the patient who is immobile.			
5. Instructs the patient to defecate into the container, or places the patient on the bedpan.			
6. Does not contaminate the specimen with toilet tissue.			
7. Explains the purpose of the test and that serial specimens may be needed.			
8. Washes hands; removes gloves.			
9. Once the specimen has been obtained, gathers the necessary testing supplies.			
10. Reads the directions for the testing kit.			
11. Dons clean procedure gloves.			
12. Opens the specimen side of the Hemoccult (or other) slide. With a wooden tongue blade or other applicator, collects a small sample of stool and spreads thinly onto one "window" of the slide.			
13. Uses a different applicator or the opposite end of the tongue blade to collect a second small sample of stool.			
14. Spreads the second sample thinly onto the second "window" of the slide.			
15. Wraps tongue blade in tissue and paper towel; places in waste receptacle. Does not flush it.			
16. Closes the Hemoccult slide.			
17. If the test is to be done by laboratory personnel, labels the specimen properly and places into the proper receptacle for transportation to the lab.			
18. If test is to be done at the bedside, turns the slide over and opens the opposite side of the package.			
19. Places one or two drops of developing solution onto each window (follows package directions).			

PROCEDURE STEPS	Yes	No	COMMENTS
20. Follows package directions for interpreting test results.			

Recommendation: Pass _____ Needs more practice _____

Student: _____ Date: _____

Instructor: _____ Date: _____

PROCEDURE CHECKLIST
Chapter 29: Performing Otic Irrigation

Check (✓) Yes or No

PROCEDURE STEPS	Yes	No	COMMENTS
1. Warms irrigating solution to body temperature (98.6°F [37.9°C]) and fills the reservoir of the irrigator.			
2. Assists the client into a sitting or lying position with the head tilted away from the affected ear.			
3. Drapes the client with a plastic drape and places a towel on the client's shoulder on the side being irrigated.			
4. Has the client hold an emesis basin under the ear to collect the irrigating fluid as it drains out of the ear. Note: An emesis basin is not necessary if a comprehensive ear wash system is used.			
5. If using an ear wash system, flushes the system to remove air. If using an Asepto or rubber bulb syringe, fills the syringe with about 50 mL of the irrigating solution and expels any remaining air.			
6. Straightens the ear canal. a. For a child less than 3 years old, pulls the pinna down and back. b. For older children and adults, pulls the pinna upward and outward.			
7. Instructs the client to indicate if any pain or dizziness occurs during the irrigation.			
8. Explains to the client that he may feel warmth, fullness, or pressure when the fluid reaches the tympanic membrane.			
9. Places the tip of the nozzle (or syringe) about 1/2 inch (1 cm) above the entrance of the ear canal and directs the stream of irrigating solution gently along the top of the ear canal toward the back of the client's head.			
10. Instills the solution slowly.			
11. Does not occlude the ear canal with the nozzle; allows the solution to flow out as it is instilled.			
12. Repeats this procedure for 5 minutes or until cerumen appears in the return solution.			
13. Inspects the ear with an otoscope to evaluate cerumen removal.			
14. Continues irrigating until the canal is cleaned.			
15. Places a cotton ball loosely in the ear canal and has the client lie on the side of the affected ear.			

PROCEDURE STEPS	Yes	No	COMMENTS

Recommendation: Pass _____ Needs more practice _____

Student: _____   Date: _____

Instructor: _____   Date: _____

PROCEDURE CHECK
Chapter 30: Connecting a Patient-Controlled Analgesia Pump

Check (✓) Yes or No

PROCEDURE STEPS	Yes	No	COMMENTS
1. Initiates IV therapy if the patient does not have an IV solution infusing.			
2. Removes air from the vial or cartridge.			
3. Connects PCA tubing to the vial or cartridge.			
4. Determines (calculates if necessary) the: a. One-time bolus (loading) dose.			
b. Basal rate.			
c. On-demand dose.			
d. Lock-out interval			
e. The 1-hour or 4-hour lock-out dosage limit.			
5. If orders are written in mg and pump settings are in mL, verifies the concentration (mg/mL) of the medication and calculates correct settings.			
6. Primes the tubing up to the Y-connector; then clamps the tubing above the connector.			
7. Inserts the container into the pump and locks the pump; or follows manufacturer's instruction manual.			
8. Turns the pump on and sets the parameters (listed in step 4, a. through e.) according to the orders and own calculations.			
9. Swabs the port on the IV tubing closest to the patient and connects the PCA pump tubing.			
10. Opens the clamp and starts the pump.			
11. Administers the bolus (loading) dose if ordered. Remains present with the patient as the dose is delivered. (To administer a loading dose, sets the pump lockout time to 0 minutes. Sets the volume to be delivered as the bolus volume calculated [e.g., if 10 mg = 0.2 mL, set the volume to 0.2 mL]; presses the button that controls the loading dose.)			
12. Closes the pump door and locks the machine with the key.			
13. Checks for flashing lights or alarms that may indicate the need to correct settings.			
14. Makes sure tubing clamps are released, and presses the start button to begin the basal infusion.			

PROCEDURE STEPS	Yes	No	COMMENTS
15. Puts the control button for on-demand doses within the patient's reach.			

Recommendation: Pass _____ Needs more practice _____

Student: _____   Date: _____

Instructor: _____   Date: _____

PROCEDURE CHECKLIST
Chapter 31: Assisting With Ambulation (One Nurse)

Check (✓)Yes or No

PROCEDURE STEPS	Yes	No	COMMENTS
1. Puts non-skid slippers on the patient.			
2. Applies a transfer belt.			
3. Places bed in low position and locks the wheels.			
4. Assists patient to dangle at the side of the bed (see checklist for Procedure Checklist Chapter 31: Dangling a Patient at the Side of the Bed).			.
5. Faces the patient. Braces feet and knees against the patient's feet and knees, paying particular attention to any known weakness.			
6. Bends the hips and knees and holds onto the transfer belt.			
7. Instructs the patient to place her arms around the nurse between the shoulders and waist (the location depends on the nurse's height and the height of the patient).			
8. Asks the patient to stand as the nurse moves to an upright position by straightening the legs and hips.			
9. Allows the patient to steady herself for a moment.			
10. Stands at the patient's side, placing both hands on the transfer belt.			
11. If the patient has weakness on one side, positions self on the weaker side.			
12. Slowly guides the patient forward, observing for signs of fatigue or dizziness.			
13. If the patient must transport an IV pole, allows the patient to hold onto the pole on the side where the nurse is standing. Assists the patient to advance the pole as they ambulate.			

Recommendation: Pass _____ Needs more practice _____

Student: _____   Date: _____

Instructor: _____   Date: _____

PROCEDURE CHECKLIST
Chapter 31: Assisting With Ambulation (Two Nurses)

Check (✓) Yes or No

PROCEDURE STEPS	Yes	No	COMMENTS
1. Puts non-skid slippers on the patient.			
2. Applies a transfer belt.			
3. Places bed in low position.			
4. Locks bed wheels.			
5. Assists patient to dangle at the side of the bed (see Procedure Checklist Chapter 31: Dangling a Patient at the Side of the Bed).			
6. Each nurse stands facing the patient on opposite sides of the patient, bracing their feet and knees against the patient's, and paying particular attention to any known weakness.			
7. Bends from the hips and knees, and holds onto the transfer belt.			
8. Instructs the patient to place her arms around each of the nurses between the shoulders and waist (the location depends on nurses' height and the height of the patient).			
9. Asks the patient to stand as the nurses move to an upright position by straightening their legs and hips.			
10. Allows patient to steady herself for a moment.			
11. Each nurse stands at the patient's sides, grasping hold of the transfer belt.			
12. Slowly guides the patient forward, observing for fatigue or dizziness.			
13. If the patient must transport an IV pole, one nurse advances the IV pole along the side of the patient by holding the pole with the outside hand.			

Recommendation: Pass _____ Needs more practice _____

Student: _____ Date: _____

Instructor: _____ Date: _____

Check (✓) Yes or No

PROCEDURE STEPS	Yes	No	COMMENTS
1. Locks bed wheels.			
2. Places patient in supine position and raises the head of the bed to 90°.			
3. Keeps side rail elevated on the side opposite where nurse is standing.			
4. Places bed in low position.			
5. Applies a gait transfer belt to the patient at waist level.			
6. Stands facing the patient with a wide base of support. Places foot closest to the head of the bed forward of the other foot. Leans forward, bending at the hips with the knees flexed.			
6. Positions hands on either side of the gait transfer belt.			
7. Rocks onto the back foot while moving the patient into a sitting position on the side of the bed—by pulling the patient by the gait transfer belt.			
8. Stays with the patient as he dangles.			

Recommendation: Pass _____ Needs more practice _____

Student: _____   Date: _____

Instructor: _____   Date: _____

PROCEDURE CHECKLIST
Chapter 31: Logrolling a Patient

Check (✓) Yes or No

PROCEDURE STEPS	Yes	No	COMMENTS
1. Locks the bed.			
2. Lowers the head of the bed and places patient supine.			
3. Ensures that a friction-reducing device such as a transfer roller sheet is in place, improvises with a plastic bag or film under patient, if needed.			
4. Lowers the side rail on the side where nurse is standing; keeps rail up on opposite side.			
5. Raises height of the bed to waist level.			
6. Positions one staff member at the patient's head and shoulders, responsible for moving the head and neck as a unit. Positions the other person at the patient's hips. If three staff members are needed, positions one at the shoulders, one at the waist, and the third at thigh level.			
7. Instructs the patient to fold her arms across her chest.			
8. Places a pillow between the patient's knees.			
9. Each nurse positions her feet with a wide base of support, with one foot slightly more forward than the other.			
10. Uses a draw sheet to move the patient to the side of the bed on which the nurses are standing.			
11. One nurse always supports the head and shoulders during the move. The move is smooth so that the head and hips are kept in alignment.			
12. Positions the patient's head with a pillow.			
13. Raises side rail and moves to opposite side of the bed.			
14. Lowers side rail on "new" side and faces the patient.			
15. All nurses position their feet with a wide base of support, with one foot forward of the other. Places weight on the forward foot.			
16. All nurses bend from the hips and position hands evenly along the length of the draw sheet.			
17. All nurses flex their knees and hips, and shift their weight to the back foot on the count of three, being sure to support head as patient is rolled.			
18. Places pillows to maintain the patient in a lateral position.			
19. Places bed in low position and raises side rails.			
20. Places call bell within reach.			

PROCEDURE STEPS	Yes	No	COMMENTS

Recommendation: Pass _____ Needs more practice _____

Student: _____   Date: _____

Instructor: _____   Date: _____

PROCEDURE CHECKLIST
Chapter 31: Moving a Patient Up In Bed

Check (✓) Yes or No

PROCEDURE STEPS	Yes	No	COMMENTS
1. Acquires second person to help with moving patient.			
2. Locks bed wheels.			
3. Lowers head of bed; places patient supine.			
4. Lowers side rail on "working" side; keeps side rail up on opposite side of the bed.			
5. Ensures that a friction-reducing device such as a transfer roller sheet is in place; improvises with a plastic bag or film under patient, if needed.			
6. Raises height of the bed to waist level.			
7. Removes pillow from under patient's head and places it at the head of the bed.			
8. Instructs the patient to fold his arms across his chest. If an overhead trapeze is in place, asks the patient to hold the trapeze with both hands. Has the patient bend his knees with feet flat on the bed.			
9. Instructs the patient to flex his neck.			
10. Positions assistant on opposite side of bed; each grasps and rolls draw sheet close to patient.			
11. Instructs the patient, on the count of three, to lift his trunk and push off with his heels toward the head of the bed.			
12. Positions own feet with a wide base of support. Points the feet toward the direction of the move. Flexes own knees and hips.			
13. Places own weight on the foot nearest to the foot of the bed. Counts to three and shifts weight forward.			
14. Repeats until the patient is positioned near the head of the bed.			
15. Straightens draw sheet, places a pillow under the patient's head and assists him to a comfortable position.			
16. Places the bed in low position, and raises the side rail.			
17. Places the call light in a position where the patient can easily reach it			

PROCEDURE STEPS	Yes	No	COMMENTS
Moving a Patient Who Is Unable to Assist or Obese			
18. Performs Steps 1 through 10.			
19. With a nurse positioned on either side of patient, uses the draw sheet to turn the patient to one side.			
20. Positions a full body sling under the patient by placing the midline at the patient's back and tucking it under the draw sheet.			
21. Turns the patient to the opposite side and unrolls the full body sling..			
22. Attaches the sling to the overbed lifting device or mechanical lift.			
23. Engages the lift to raise the patient off of the bed. Advances the lift toward the head of the bed until the patient is at the desired level.			
24. Lowers the lift and removes sling from underneath patient, if needed.			
25. Turns patient to the desired position. Straightens the draw sheet and tucks it in tightly at the sides of the bed.			

Recommendation: Pass _____ Needs more practice _____

Student: _____   Date: _____

Instructor: _____   Date: _____

PROCEDURE CHECKLIST
Chapter 31: Transferring a Patient from Bed to Chair

Check (✓) Yes or No

PROCEDURE STEPS	Yes	No	COMMENTS
1. Positions the chair next to the bed and near the head of the bed. If possible, locks the chair.			
2. Puts non-skid slippers on the patient.			
3. Applies the transfer belt.			
4. Places bed in low position.			
5. Locks the bed.			
6. Assists patient to dangle at the side of the bed (see Procedure Checklist Chapter 31: Dangling a Patient at the Side of the Bed).			
7. Faces the patient; braces feet and knees against the patient's feet and knees. Pays particular attention to any known weakness.			
8. Bends hips and knees; holds onto the transfer belt. If two nurses are available, one nurse should be on each side of the patient.			
9. Instructs the patient to place her arms around the nurse between the shoulders and waist (the exact location depends on the height of the nurse and patient).			
10. Asks patient to stand as the nurse moves to an upright position by straightening her legs and hips.			
11. Allows the patient to steady herself for a moment.			
12. Instructs the patient to pivot and turn with the nurse toward the chair.			
13. Assists the patient to position herself in front of the chair and place her hands on the arms of the chair.			
14. Has the patient flex her hips and knees as she lowers herself to the chair. Guides her motion while maintaining a firm hold of the patient.			
15. Assists the patient to a comfortable position in the chair.			

Recommendation: Pass _____ Needs more practice _____

Student: _____   Date: _____

Instructor: _____   Date: _____

Check (✓) Yes or No

PROCEDURE STEPS	Yes	No	COMMENTS
1. Locks the bed.			
2. Positions the bed flat (if the patient can tolerate being supine) and at the height of the stretcher.			
3. Lowers the side rails.			
4. Positions at least one nurse on each side of the bed.			
5. Moves the patient to the side of the bed where the stretcher will be placed by rolling up the draw sheet close to the patient's body and pulling.			
6. Aligns the patient's legs and head with her trunk.			
7. Positions stretcher next to the bed.			
8. Locks stretcher.			
9. Nurse on the side of the bed opposite the stretcher uses draw sheet to turn the client away from the stretcher; the other nurse places the transfer board with a friction-reducing device such as a transfer roller sheet against the patient's back, halfway between the bed and the stretcher.			
10. Uses draw sheet to slide the patient across the transfer board onto the stretcher.			
11. Turns the patient away from the bed and removes the board and transfer roller sheet.			
12. Repositions patient on the stretcher for comfort and alignment; provides a blanket if needed.			
13. Fastens safety belts and raises stretcher side rails.			
Variation: Transferring from Bed to Stretcher with a Slipsheet			
14. Follows steps 1 through 4 above.			
15. Nurse on the side of the bed opposite the stretcher uses draw sheet to turn the client away from the stretcher; the other nurse positions the midline of the slip sheet under the patient. Rolls the remaining half tightly and tucks under patient.			
16. Turns the patient to the opposite side and pulls the slip sheet from under the patient.			
17. Lowers the side rail on the side where the stretcher will be placed.			

PROCEDURE STEPS	Yes	No	COMMENTS
18. Positions the stretcher next to the bed and locks the wheels.			
19. Positions at least two nurses on the far side of the stretcher. Pulls the patient onto the stretcher by pulling on the slip sheet.			
20. Follows steps 11 through 13 above.			

Recommendation: Pass _____ Needs more practice _____

Student: _____   Date: _____

Instructor: _____   Date: _____

PROCEDURE CHECKLIST
Chapter 31: Turning a Patient in Bed

Check (✓) Yes or No

PROCEDURE STEPS	Yes	No	COMMENTS
1. Acquires second person to help with turning.			
2. Locks the bed.			
3. Lowers the head of the bed and places patient supine.			
4. Positions self and assistant on opposite sides of the bed.			
5. Lowers the side rails.			
6. Ensures that a friction-reducing device such as a transfer roller sheet is in place; improvises with a plastic bag or film under patient, if needed.			
7. Raises height of the bed to waist level.			
8. Moves the patient to the side of the bed he is turning him away from by rolling up the draw sheet close to the patient's body and pulling.			
9. Aligns the patient's legs and head with his trunk.			
10. Places the patient's near leg and foot across the far leg (e.g., when turning right, places left leg over right).			
11. Places the patient's near arm across his chest. Abducts and externally rotates the other arm and shoulder.			
12. Stands with a wide base of support with one foot forward of the other.			
13. Grasps draw sheet at level of shoulders and hips. .			
14. Places weight on the forward foot.			
15. Bends from the hips and knees.			
16. Instructs the patient that the turn will occur on the count of three.			
17. If positioned on the side toward which the patient will turn, flexes own knees and hips and shifts weight to the back foot while pulling on the draw sheet at the hip and shoulder level, If positioned on the opposite side, shifts weight forward.			
18. Positions patient's dependent shoulder forward.			
19. Places pillows to maintain patient in lateral position.			
20. Places the bed in low position and raises the side rails.			
21. Places the call light in easy reach.			

PROCEDURE STEPS	Yes	No	COMMENTS

Recommendation: Pass _____ Needs more practice _____

Student: _____   Date: _____

Instructor: _____   Date: _____

Check (✓) Yes or No

PROCEDURE STEPS	Yes	No	COMMENTS
1. Warms the lotion in warm water.			
2. Raises bed to working height.			
3. Positions patient comfortably on side or prone; keeps side rail raised on opposite side of the bed.			
4. Unties patient's gown and exposes back.			
5. Washes patient's back with warm water if needed.			
6. Puts lotions on own hands.			
7. Places hands on either side of the spine at the base of the neck; using a gentle, continuous pressure, rubs down the length of the spine and then up the sides of the back. Repeats several times.			
8. Does not rub directly over the spine.			
9. Next, applies gentle thumb pressure on either side of the spine at mid-back, pushing outward for about an inch. Repeats from the mid-back to the base of the neck in a series of small, outward strokes.			
10. Always applies pressure away from the spine, not toward it.			
11. Asks patient if the amount of pressure is comfortable.			
12. If unable to do both sides of the spine at the same time, does one and then the other.			
13. Next, moves to the spots that felt the tightest or that the patient states are tight, and works in small circles, using gentle thumb pressure.			
14. Using palm of hand, gently shakes one scapula and then the other.			
15. Using horizontal strokes from near the spine across the bottom of the scapula, pushes out all the way across the scapula from the spine. Moves up and repeats until the entire scapula and top of shoulder have been covered.			
16. If tender spots are located, applies pressure using the fleshy parts of the fingers in a small circular motion.			
17. Begins at the upper shoulder and works down to the lower back, applying pressure in medium-sized circles down each side of the spine with the heels of the hands.			

PROCEDURE STEPS	Yes	No	COMMENTS
18. Takes care not to apply too much pressure; assesses patient for comfort.			
19. Next, using horizontal strokes from near the spine below the scapula, pushes out from the spine across to the ribs and works down across the lower back with heels of hands.			
20. With long strokes, gently rubs hands up both sides of the spine from the base of the back to the base of the neck, and then down the sides of the back. Repeats several times.			
21. If unable to do a complete back massage, asks patient where he is most uncomfortable and massages those areas. If the patient has general tightness, uses long strokes down each side of the spine and back up the sides.			

Recommendation: Pass _____ Needs more practice _____

Student: _____   Date: _____

Instructor: _____   Date: _____

PROCEDURE CHECKLIST
Chapter 34: Applying a Hydrocolloid Dressing

Check (✓) Yes or No

PROCEDURE STEPS	Yes	No	COMMENTS
1. Places the patient in a comfortable position that provides easy access to the wound.			
2. If a dressing is present, washes hands, applies clean gloves, and removes the old dressing.			
3. Disposes of the soiled dressing and gloves in the biohazard waste.			
4. Washes hands. Applies clean gloves.			
5. Cleanses the skin surrounding the wound with normal saline or a mild cleansing agent. Rinses the skin well if a cleanser is used.			
6. Allows the skin to dry.			
7. Does not attempt to remove residue that is left on the skin from the old dressing.			
8. Cleanses the wound as ordered.			
9. Uses clean or sterile technique, depending on the type of wound.			
10. Assesses the condition of the wound; notes the size, location, type of tissue present, amount of exudate, and odor.			
11. Removes soiled gloves; disposes appropriately.			
12. With backing still intact, cuts the hydrocolloid dressing to the desired shape and size. The hydrocolloid dressing should extend 3–4 cm (1.5 inches) beyond the wound margin on all sides.			
13. Applies clean gloves.			
14. Removes the backing of the hydrocolloid dressing, starting at one edge. Places the exposed adhesive portion on the patient's skin.			
15. Positions the dressing to provide coverage of the wound.			
16. Gradually peels away the remaining liner and smoothes the hydrocolloid dressing onto the skin by placing a hand on top of the dressing and holding in place for 1 minute.			
17. Assists patient to a comfortable position and removes gloves.			
18. Washes hands.			

PROCEDURE STEPS	Yes	No	COMMENTS

Recommendation: Pass _____ Needs more practice _____

Student: _____   Date: _____

Instructor: _____   Date: _____

PROCEDURE CHECKLIST
Chapter 34: Applying a Transparent Film Dressing

Check (✓) Yes or No

PROCEDURE STEPS	Yes	No	COMMENTS
1. Places the patient in a comfortable position that provides easy access to the wound.			
2. If a dressing is present, washes hands, applies clean gloves, and removes the old dressing.			
3. Disposes of the soiled dressing and gloves in the biohazard waste.			
4. Applies clean gloves and cleanses the skin surrounding the wound with normal saline or a mild cleansing agent. Rinses the skin well if a cleanser is used.			
5. Allows the skin to dry.			
6. If hair is present in the area where the dressing will be applied, clips the hair with scissors.			
7. If the skin is oily, cleans the surrounding skin with alcohol or acetone and allows it to dry.			
8. Cleanses the wound as ordered or according to agency procedure.			
9. Correctly uses clean or sterile technique, depending on the nature of the wound.			
10. Assesses the condition of the wound. Notes the size, location, type of tissue present, amount of exudate, and odor.			
11. Removes the center backing liner from the transparent film dressing.			
12. Holding the dressing by the edges, applies the transparent film to the wound. Maintains a slight stretch on the edges of the dressing when applying to prevent wrinkling.			
13. Removes the edging liner from the dressing.			
14. Properly disposes of soiled equipment and removes gloves.			

Recommendation: Pass _____ Needs more practice _____

Student: _____   Date: _____

Instructor: _____   Date: _____

Check (✓) Yes or No

PROCEDURE STEPS	Yes	No	COMMENTS
1. Administers pain medication 30 minutes prior to procedure, if necessary.			
2. Positions the patient so the wound is easily accessible.			
3. Positions a water-resistant disposable drape under the patient to collect fluid runoff.			
4. After washing and drying hands, applies a gown, face shield, and clean gloves.			
5. Removes the soiled dressing. Disposes of gloves and soiled dressing in a biohazard bag.			
6. Sets up a sterile field using an impermeable barrier on the bedside table.			
7. Opens packets of sterile 4×4 gauze onto the field. Moistens the gauze with 0.9% (normal) saline solution for irrigation.			
8. As an alternative to setting up a sterile field (Steps 6 and 7), may use an impermeable tray of sterile 4×4 gauze. Removes the cover of the tray and moistens the gauze with sterile saline.			
9. Attaches a 22 gauge needle to a 3 mL syringe and withdraws 1 mL of sterile 0.9% saline for injection from the vial.			
10. Caps the needle, using a one-handed technique (see Procedure Checklist Chapter 23: Recapping Needles Using One-Handed Technique) and places it on the bedside table.			
11. Applies sterile gloves.			
12. Gently cleanses the wound with the saline moistened gauze by lightly wiping a section of the wound from the center toward the wound edge.			
13. Discards the gauze in a biohazard receptacle and repeats in the next section using a new piece of gauze with each wiping pass.			
14. Uncaps the syringe from the bedside table and inserts the needle 1 to 2 mm into the wound bed.			

PROCEDURE STEPS	Yes	No	COMMENTS
15. Injects 1 mL of 0.9% saline into the wound tissue.			
16. Pulls back on the syringe plunger to aspirate approximately 1 mL of fluid into the barrel of the syringe. Removes the needle from the wound bed after collecting the aspirate.			
17. Places the collected fluid into a culture tube containing culture medium.			
18. Labels the culture tube with the patient's name, birthdate, source of specimen, and date and time of collection. (A label may be supplied with the culture kit.)			
19. Transports the culture to the lab.			
20. Applies a clean dressing to the wound as ordered.			

Recommendation: Pass _____ Needs more practice _____

Student: _____   Date: _____

Instructor: _____   Date: _____

Check (✓) Yes or No

PROCEDURE STEPS	Yes	No	COMMENTS
1. Places the patient in a comfortable position that provides easy access to the wound and will allow the irrigation solution to flow freely from the wound, with the assistance of gravity.			
2. Places a water-resistant disposable drape to protect the bedding from any runoff.			
3. After washing and drying the hands, applies a gown, face shield, and clean gloves.			
4. Removes the soiled dressing. Disposes of gloves and soiled dressing in a biohazard bag.			
5. Applies clean gloves.			
6. Places an emesis basin at the bottom of the wound to collect irrigation runoff.			
7. Avoids touching the wound with the basin.			
8. Attaches a 19 gauge Angiocath to a 35 cc syringe and fills it with normal saline irrigation solution.			
9. Holding the Angiocath tip 2 cm from the wound bed, gently irrigates the wound with a back and forth motion, moving from the superior aspect to the inferior aspect.			
10. Disposes of the syringe and Angiocath in the sharps container, and gloves in the biohazard waste.			
11. Obtains a Culturette tube and twists the top of the tube to loosen the swab.			
12. Applies clean gloves and locates an area of red, granulating tissue in the wound bed.			
13. Withdraws the swab from the Culturette tube. Presses the swab against the granulating area and rotates the swab.			
a. Does not allow the swab to touch anything other than the granulating area of the wound.			
b. Does not swab culture areas with slough or eschar present.			

PROCEDURE STEPS	Yes	No	COMMENTS
14. Carefully inserts the swab back into the Culturette tube, making sure it does not make contact with the opening of tube upon reinsertion.			
15. Twists the cap to secure the tube.			
16. Crushes the ampule of culture medium at the bottom of the tube. (Note: Inspects the culture tube used to determine if this step is required.)			
17. Labels the Culturette tube with the patient's name, birthdate, source of specimen, and date and time of collection. (Labels may be provided with the Culturette kit.)			
18. Applies a clean dressing to the wound as ordered.			

Recommendation: Pass _____ Needs more practice _____

Student: _____   Date: _____

Instructor: _____   Date: _____

Check (✓) Yes or No

PROCEDURE STEPS	Yes	No	COMMENTS
1. Administers pain medication 30 minutes prior to procedure, if necessary.			
2. Warms irrigation solution.			
3. Places the patient in a comfortable position that provides easy access to the wound and will allow the irrigation solution to flow freely from the wound, with the assistance of gravity.			
4. Positions a water-resistant disposable drape to protect the bedding from any possible runoff.			
5. After washing and drying hands, applies a gown, face shield, and clean gloves.			
6. Removes the soiled dressing. Disposes of gloves and soiled dressing in a biohazard bag.			
7. Sets up a sterile field on a clean dry surface.			
8. Adds the following supplies to the field: 　　Sterile gauze 　　Sterile bowl 　　Dressing supplies 　　Variation A: A 19 gauge Angiocath, 35 cc 　　　syringe, and sterile emesis basin, or 　　Variation B: A sterile commercial irrigation 　　　kit			
9. Pours the warmed irrigation solution into the sterile bowl.			
10. Dons sterile gloves.			
11. Irrigates the wound. 　a. Places the sterile emesis basin at the bottom of the wound to collect irrigation runoff.			
b. Variation A: Attaches the 19 gauge Angiocath to the 35 mL syringe and fills with the irrigation solution, or 　　Variation B: Fills a piston-tip or bulb syringe with irrigation solution.			

PROCEDURE STEPS	Yes	No	COMMENTS
c. Holding the Angiocath tip or syringe tip 2 cm from the wound bed, gently irrigates the wound with a back and forth motion, moving from the superior aspect to the inferior aspect.			
d. Repeats the irrigation until the solution returns clear.			
12. Removes the basin or sterile container from the base of the wound; pats the skin around the wound dry with sterile gauze, beginning at the top of the wound and working downward.			
13. Dresses the wound as ordered.			
14. Disposes of contaminated irrigation fluid in an appropriate manner (biohazardous waste).			
15. Removes soiled drapes from the patient area.			
16. Removes gloves, face shield, and gown; disposes of appropriately (they are biohazardous).			
17. Washes hands.			
18. Repositions patient to a comfortable position.			

Recommendation: Pass _____ Needs more practice _____

Student: _____ Date: _____

Instructor: _____ Date: _____

PROCEDURE CHECKLIST
Chapter 34: Removing and Applying Dry Dressings

Check (✓) Yes or No

PROCEDURE STEPS	Yes	No	COMMENTS
Removing Old Dressing and Cleansing Wound			
1. Places the patient in a comfortable position that provides easy access to the wound.			
2. Washes hands and applies clean gloves.			
3. Loosens the edges of the tape of the old dressing. Stabilizes the skin with one hand while pulling the tape in the opposite direction.			
4. Beginning at the edges of the dressing, lifts the dressing toward the center of the wound.			
5. If the dressing sticks, moistens it with 0.9% (normal) saline before completely removing it.			
6. Assesses the type and amount of drainage present on the soiled dressing.			
7. Disposes of soiled dressing and gloves in a biohazard bag.			
8. Removes the cover of a tray of sterile 4×4 gauze. Moistens the gauze with sterile saline.			
9. Applies clean gloves.			
10. Gently cleanses the wound with the saline-moistened gauze by lightly wiping a section of the wound from the center toward the wound edge.			
11. Discards the gauze in a biohazard receptacle and repeats in the next section, using a new piece of gauze with each wiping pass.			
12. Discards gloves and soiled gauze into a biohazard bag.			
Applying the Dry Dressing			
1. Washes hands.			
2. Opens sterile gauze packages on a clean, dry surface.			
3. Applies clean gloves.			
4. Applies a layer of dry dressings over the wound; if drainage is expected, uses an additional layer of dressings.			
5. Removes gloves, turning them inside out, and discards in a biohazard receptacle.			

PROCEDURE STEPS	Yes	No	COMMENTS
6. Places strips of tape at the ends of the dressing and evenly spaced over the remainder of the dressing. Uses strips that are sufficiently long to secure the dressing in place.			

Recommendation: Pass _____ Needs more practice _____

Student: _____ Date: _____

Instructor: _____ Date: _____

PROCEDURE CHECKLIST
Chapter 34: Removing and Applying Wet-to-Damp Dressings

Check (✓) Yes or No

PROCEDURE STEPS	Yes	No	COMMENTS
Removing the Soiled Dressing			
1. Assesses for pain and medicates 30 minutes prior to procedure, if needed.			
2. Places the patient in a comfortable position that provides easy access to the wound.			
3. Washes hands and applies clean gloves.			
4. Loosens the edges of the tape of the old dressing. Stabilizes the skin with the other hand while pulling the tape in the opposite direction.			
5. Beginning with the top layer, lifts the dressing from the corner toward the center of the wound. If dressing sticks, moistens with 0.9% (normal) saline before completely removing it.			
6. Continues to remove layers until the entire dressing is removed.			
7. Assesses the type and amount of drainage present on the soiled dressing.			
8. Disposes of soiled dressing and gloves in a biohazard bag.			
9. Removes the cover of a tray of sterile 4×4 gauze; moistens the gauze with sterile saline.			
10. Applies clean gloves.			
11. Gently cleanses the wound with the saline-moistened gauze by lightly wiping a section of the wound from the center toward the wound edge.			
12. Discards the gauze in a biohazard receptacle and repeats in the next section using a new piece of gauze with each wiping pass.			
13. Discards gloves and soiled gauze into a biohazard bag.			
Procedural Steps for Applying Wet-to-Damp Dressing			
14. Establishes a sterile field, using a sterile impermeable barrier.			
15. Opens sterile gauze packs and a surgipad onto the sterile field. The amount of gauze used will depend on the size of the wound.			
16. Moistens sterile gauze with a sterile 0.9% saline solution for irrigation.			
17. Applies clean gloves.			

PROCEDURE STEPS	Yes	No	COMMENTS
18. Wrings out excess moisture from the gauze before applying.			
19. Applies a single layer of moist fine-mesh gauze to the wound, being careful to place gauze in all depressions or crevices of the wound. Uses sterile forceps or cotton applicator to ensure that deep depressions or sinus tracts are filled with gauze.			
20. Applies a secondary moist layer over the first layer. Repeats this process until the wound is completely filled with moistened sterile gauze.			
21. Does not pack the gauze tightly into the wound.			
22. Does not extend the moist dressing onto the surrounding skin.			
23. Covers the moistened gauze with a surgipad.			
24. Secures the dressing with tape or Montgomery straps.			
25. Disposes of gloves and sterile field materials in the biohazard waste.			

Recommendation: Pass _____ Needs more practice _____

Student: _____   Date: _____

Instructor: _____   Date: _____

PROCEDURE CHECKLIST
Chapter 35: Administering Oxygen by Cannula, Face Mask, or Face Tent

Check (✓) Yes or No

PROCEDURE STEPS	Yes	No	COMMENTS
1. Attaches the flow meter to the wall oxygen source. If using a portable oxygen tank, attaches the flow meter to the tank if it is not already connected.			
2. Assembles and applies the oxygen equipment.			
Variation: Nasal Cannula			
3. Attaches the humidifier to the flow meter. (Humidification is only necessary for flow rates of > 3 LPM.) If a humidifier is not used, attaches the adapter to the flow meter.			
4. Attaches the nasal cannula to the humidifier or the adapter.			
5. Places the nasal prongs in the patient's nares, then places the tubing around each ear.			
6. Uses the slide adjustment device to tighten the cannula under the patient's chin.			
7. Turns on the oxygen, using the flow meter, and adjusts it according to the prescribed flow rate.			
8. Makes sure that the oxygen equipment is set up correctly and functioning properly before leaving the patient's bedside.			
Variation: Face Mask			
9. Attaches the prefilled humidifier to the flow meter.			
10. Attaches the oxygen tubing from the mask to the humidifier.			
11. Gently places the face mask on the patient's face, applying it from the bridge of the nose to under the chin.			
12. Secures the elastic band around the back of the patient's head, making sure the mask fits snugly but comfortably.			
13. Turns on the oxygen, using the flow meter, and adjusts it according to the prescribed flow rate.			
14. Makes sure that the oxygen equipment is set up correctly and functioning properly before leaving the patient's bedside.			
Variation: Face Tent			
15. Attaches the prefilled humidifier to the flow meter.			
16. Attaches the oxygen tubing to the face tent.			

PROCEDURE STEPS	Yes	No	COMMENTS
17. Attaches the oxygen tubing to the humidifier.			
18. Gently places the face tent in front of the patient's face, making sure that it fits under the chin.			
19. Secures the elastic band around the back of the patient's head.			
20. Turns on the oxygen using the flow meter and adjusts it according to the prescribed flow rate.			
21. Makes sure that the oxygen equipment is set up correctly and functioning properly before leaving the patient's bedside.			

Recommendation: Pass _____ Needs more practice _____

Student: _____   Date: _____

Instructor: _____   Date: _____

PROCEDURE CHECKLIST
Chapter 35: Applying and Caring for a Patient with a Cardiac Monitor

Check (✓) Yes or No

PROCEDURE STEPS	Yes	No	COMMENTS
1. For hardwire monitoring: Plugs the monitor into an electrical outlet and turns it on. Connects the cable with lead wires into the monitor. For Telemetry Monitoring: Inserts a new battery into the transmitter; turns on the transmitter; connects the lead wires to the transmitter (if not permanently attached), taking care to attach each one to its correct outlet.			
2. Exposes the patient's chest and identifies electrode sites based on the monitoring system being used and the patient's anatomy.			
3. If the patient's chest contains dense hair, shaves or clips the hair with scissors at each electrode site.			
4. Cleans the areas chosen for electrode placement with an alcohol pad; allows them to dry.			
5. Gently rubs the placement sites with a washcloth or gauze pad until the skin reddens slightly.			
6. Removes the electrode backing and makes sure the gel is moist. Applies the electrodes to the sites by pressing firmly.			
7. Attaches the lead wires to the electrodes by snapping or clipping them in place.			
8. Secures the monitoring equipment. For hardwire monitoring: Wraps a piece of 1-inch tape around the cable and secures it to the patient's gown with a safety pin. For telemetry monitoring: Places the transmitter in the pouch and ties the pouch strings around the patient's neck and waist. Places the transmitter into the patient's robe pocket if a pouch is not available.			
9. Checks the patient's ECG tracing on the monitor. If necessary, adjusts the gain on the monitor to increase the waveform size.			
10. Sets the upper and lower heart rate alarm limits according to agency policy or patient's condition and turns them on.			
11. Obtains a rhythm strip by pressing the "record" button. For hardwire monitoring: Presses the "record" button on the bedside monitor.			

PROCEDURE STEPS	Yes	No	COMMENTS
<u>For telemetry monitoring</u>: Presses the "record" button on the transmitter of the telemetry unit.			
12. Interprets the rhythm strip and mounts it appropriately (e.g., with transparent tape) in the patient's chart.			

<u>Recommendation</u>: Pass _____ Needs more practice _____

Student: _____   Date: _____

Instructor: _____   Date: _____

PROCEDURE CHECKLIST
Chapter 35: Caring for a Patient on a Mechanical Ventilator

Check (✓) Yes or No

PROCEDURE STEPS	Yes	No	COMMENTS
1. Prepares a resuscitation bag: Attaches a flow meter to one of the oxygen sources; attaches an adapter to the flow meter; and connects the oxygen tubing to the adapter.			
2. The respiratory therapy department is responsible for setting up mechanical ventilators in most agencies. If necessary to assume the responsibility, refers to the manufacturer's instructions.			
3. Verifies ventilator settings with the physician's order.			
4. Checks the ventilator alarm limits. Makes sure they are set appropriately.			
5. Attaches the ventilator tubing to the endotracheal or tracheostomy tube.			
6. Places the ventilator tubing in the securing device.			
7. Prepares the suction equipment (see Checklist Procedure Checklist Chapter 35: Performing Tracheostomy or Endotracheal Suctioning).			
8. Checks the ventilator tubing frequently for condensation.			
9. Drains the fluid into a collection device or briefly disconnects the patient from the ventilator and empties the tubing into a waste receptacle, according to agency policy.			
10. Never drains the fluid into the humidifier.			
11. Checks ventilator settings regularly.			
12. Provides the patient with an alternate form of communication, such as a letter board or white board.			
13. Repositions regularly, being careful not to pull on the ventilator tubing.			
14. Provides frequent oral care, moistens the lips with a cool, damp cloth and water-based lubricant.			
15. Ensures that the call light is always within reach and answers call light and ventilator alarms promptly.			

PROCEDURE STEPS	Yes	No	COMMENTS

Recommendation: Pass _____ Needs more practice _____

Student: _____   Date: _____

Instructor: _____   Date: _____

Check (✓) Yes or No

PROCEDURE STEPS	Yes	No	COMMENTS
1. Obtains and prepares the prescribed drainage system.			
a. <u>Disposable water-seal system without suction.</u> 1) Removes the cover on the water-seal chamber and, using the funnel provided, fills the second (water-seal) chamber with sterile water or normal saline. Fills to the 2-cm mark, or as indicated. 2) Replaces the cover on the water-seal chamber.			
b. <u>Disposable water-seal system with suction.</u> 1) Removes the cover on the water-seal chamber and, using the funnel provided, fills the water-seal chamber (second chamber) with sterile water or normal saline to the 2-cm mark.			
2) Adds sterile water or normal saline solution to the suction-control chamber. Adds the amount of fluid specified by the physician order, typically 20 cm.			
3) Attaches the tubing from the suction-control chamber to the connecting tubing attached to the suction source.			
2. Positions the patient according to the indicated insertion site.			
3. Dons a mask, gown, and sterile gloves.			
4. Provides support to the patient while the physician prepares the sterile field, anesthetizes the patient, and inserts and sutures the chest tube.			
5. As soon as the chest tube is inserted, attaches it to drainage system using a connector.			
6. Using sterile technique, wraps petroleum gauze around the chest tube insertion site.			
7. Places a precut, sterile drain dressing over the petroleum gauze.			
8. Places a second sterile, precut, drain dressing over the first drain dressing with the opening facing in the opposite direction from the first one.			
9. Places a large drainage dressing ("ABD") over the two precut drain dressings.			
10. Secures the dressing in place with 2-inch silk tape, making sure to cover the dressing completely.			

PROCEDURE STEPS	Yes	No	COMMENTS
11. Writes date, time, and initials on the dressing.			
12. Using the spiral taping technique, wraps 1-inch silk tape around the chest tube starting above the connector and continuing below the connector. Reverses the wrapping by taping back up the tubing (using the spiral technique) until above the connector.			
13. Cuts an 8-inch-long piece of 2-inch tape. Loops one end around the top portion of the drainage tube and secures the remaining end of the tape to the chest tube dressing.			
14. If suction is prescribed, adjusts the suction source until gentle bubbling occurs in the suction-control chamber. If suction is not prescribed, leaves the suction tubing on the drainage system open.			
15. Makes sure that the drainage tubing lies with no kinks from the chest tube to the drainage chamber.			
16. Prepares the patient for a portable chest x-ray.			
17. Places two rubber-tipped clamps at the patient's bedside for special situations (safety measure).			
18. Places a petroleum gauze dressing at the bedside in case the chest tube becomes dislodged.			
19. Keeps a spare disposable drainage system at the patient's bedside.			
20. Positions patient for comfort, as indicated.			
21. Maintains chest tube and drainage system patency by: a. Making sure the drainage tubing is free of kinks.			
b. Inspecting the air vent in the drainage system to make sure it is patent.			
c. Making sure the drainage system is located below the insertion site.			

Recommendation: Pass _____ Needs more practice _____

Student: _____   Date: _____

Instructor: _____   Date: _____

PROCEDURE CHECKLIST
Chapter 35: Collecting an Expectorated Specimen

Check (✓) Yes or No

PROCEDURE STEPS	Yes	No	COMMENTS
1. Positions patient in a high or semi-Fowler's position, or sitting on the edge of the bed.			
2. Drapes a towel or linen-saver pad over the patient's chest.			
3. If the patient has an abdominal or chest incision, has the patient splint the incision with a pillow.			
4. Hands the patient a glass of water and an emesis basin and has him rinse his mouth.			
5. Provides the patient with the specimen container. Advises the patient to avoid touching the inside of the container.			
6. Asks the patient to breathe deeply for three or four breaths, and then asks him after a full inhalation, to hold his breath, and then cough.			
7. Instructs the patient to expectorate the secretions directly into the specimen container.			
8. Tells the patient to repeat deep breathing and coughing until an adequate sample is obtained.			
9. Covers the specimen container with the lid immediately after the specimen is collected.			
10. Labels the specimen container with a patient identification label that contains the name of the test and collection date and time.			
11. Places the specimen in a plastic bag labeled with a biohazard label. Attaches a completed laboratory requisition form.			
12. Sends the specimen immediately to the laboratory, or refrigerates it if transport might be delayed.			

Recommendation: Pass _____ Needs more practice _____

Student: _____   Date: _____

Instructor: _____   Date: _____

PROCEDURE CHECKLIST
Chapter 35: Collecting a Suctioned Specimen

Check (✓) Yes or No

PROCEDURE STEPS	Yes	No	COMMENTS
1. Positions patient in a high or semi-Fowler's position.			
2. Drapes a towel or linen-saver pad over the patient's chest.			
3. If the patient has an abdominal or chest incision, has the patient splint the incision with a pillow.			
4. Administers oxygen to the patient, if indicated.			
5. Prepares the suction device and makes sure it is functioning properly.			
6. Dons protective eye wear.			
7. Attaches the suction tubing to the male adapter of the inline sputum specimen container.			
8. Dons sterile gloves.			
9. Attaches the sterile suction catheter to the rubber tubing of the inline sputum specimen container.			
10. Lubricates the suction catheter with sterile saline solution.			
11. Inserts the tip of the suction catheter gently through the nasopharynx, endotracheal tube, or tracheostomy tube and advances it into the trachea. (See Procedure Checklist Chapter 35: Performing Tracheostomy Care or Procedure Checklist Chapter 35: Performing Oropharyngeal and Nasopharyngeal Suctioning.).			
12. When the patient begins coughing, applies suction for 5 to 10 seconds to collect the specimen.			
13. If an adequate specimen (5 to 10 mL) is not obtained, allows the patient to rest for 1 minute and then repeats the procedure. Administers oxygen to the patient at this time, if indicated.			

PROCEDURE STEPS	Yes	No	COMMENTS
14. When an adequate specimen is collected, discontinues suction, then gently removes the suction catheter.			
15. Removes the suction catheter from the specimen container and disposes of the catheter in the appropriate container.			
16. Removes the suction tubing from the specimen container and connects the rubber tubing on the specimen container to the plastic adapter.			
17. If sputum comes in contact with the outside of the specimen container, cleans it with a disinfectant according to agency policy.			
18. Labels the specimen container with a patient identification label that contains the name of the test and collection date and time.			
19. Sends the specimen to the laboratory immediately or refrigerates it if transport might be delayed.			

Recommendation: Pass _____ Needs more practice _____

Student: _____   Date: _____

Instructor: _____   Date: _____

PROCEDURE CHECKLIST
Chapter 35: Monitoring Pulse Oximetry (Arterial Oxygen Saturation)

Check (✓) Yes or No

PROCEDURE STEPS	Yes	No	COMMENTS
1. Chooses a sensor appropriate for the patient's age, size, and weight; and the desired location.			
2. If the patient is allergic to adhesive, uses a clip-on probe sensor. Uses a nasal sensor if the patient's peripheral circulation is compromised.			
3. Prepares the site by cleansing and drying.			
4. If the finger is the desired monitoring location, removes nail polish or an acrylic nail, if present.			
5. Removes the protective backing if using a disposable probe sensor that contains adhesive.			
6. Attaches the probe sensor to the chosen site. Makes sure that the photo-detector and light-emitting diodes on the probe sensor face each other.			
7. If a clip-on probe sensor is used, warns the patient that he may feel a pinching sensation.			
8. Connects the sensor probe to the oximeter and turns it on.			
9. Checks the pulse rate displayed on the oximeter to see if it correlates with the patient's radial pulse.			
10. Reads the SaO_2 measurement on the digital display when it reaches a constant value, usually in 10 to 30 seconds.			
11. Sets and turns on the alarm limits for SaO_2 and pulse rate, according to manufacturer instructions, patient condition, and agency policy, if continuous monitoring is necessary.			
12. Obtains readings as ordered or indicated by the patient's respiratory status.			
13. Rotates the probe site every 4 hours for an adhesive probe sensor and every 2 hours for a clip-on probe sensor, if continuous monitoring is indicated.			
14. Removes the probe sensor and turns off the oximeter when monitoring is no longer necessary.			

Recommendation: Pass _____ Needs more practice _____

Student: _____ Date: _____

Instructor: _____ Date: _____

PROCEDURE CHECKLIST
Chapter 35: Performing Cardiopulmonary Resuscitation, One- and Two-Person

We have intentionally <u>not</u> provided a checklist for this procedure because students should be certified in CPR, using official tests and materials. As a quick review, but not as a "check-off," you can use the critical aspects, that follow:

Critical Aspects

- Establish whether the patient is unresponsive (shake and shout, "Are you OK?")
- Activate the emergency response system immediately if the patient is an adult. If you are alone and the patient is an infant or child, perform CPR for 1 minute then activate the emergency response system.
- Carefully place the patient on a hard surface. Logroll the patient if a cervical spine injury is suspected. If the patient is in a hospital bed, place a CPR board under the patient's back.
- Properly position yourself.
- *A—Airway.* Open the patient's airway. Use either the head tilt-chin lift maneuver or the jaw thrust maneuver.
- *B—Breathing.* Check for breathing. (Place your ear over the patient's mouth and nose. Look, listen, and feel for breathing for no longer than 10 seconds.) If the patient is breathing, continue to hold the airway open. If the patient is not breathing, administer 2 slow breaths.
- *C—Circulation.* Check for signs of circulation. Use the carotid pulse in adults and children, and the brachial or femoral pulse in infants. Assess for a pulse for 5 to 10 seconds. Also check for other signs of circulation, such as movement.
- If signs of circulation are absent, correctly position your hands and begin chest compressions.
- Continue CPR for 4 cycles then reassess pulse.

Stop CPR if the patient responds, regains an adequate pulse and begins to breathe, you are too exhausted to continue; or signs of death are obvious.

<u>Recommendation</u>: Pass _____ Needs more practice _____

Student: _____ Date: _____

Instructor: _____ Date: _____

PROCEDURE CHECKLIST
Chapter 35: Performing Nasotracheal Suctioning

Check (✓) Yes or No

PROCEDURE STEPS	Yes	No	COMMENTS
1. Positions the patient in semi-Fowler's position with his head hyperextended, unless contraindicated.			
2. Places the linen-saver pad or towel on the patient's chest.			
3. Puts on a face shield or goggles.			
4. Turns on the wall suction or portable suction machine and adjusts the pressure regulator according to agency policy (typically 100 to 120 mm Hg for adults, 95 to 110 mm Hg for children, and 50 to 95 mm Hg for infants).			
5. Tests the suction equipment by occluding the connection tubing.			
6. Opens the suction catheter kit or the gathered equipment if a kit isn't available. Opens the water-soluble lubricant.			
7. Dons sterile gloves (alternatively, puts a sterile glove on the dominant hand and a clean procedure glove on the nondominant hand); considers the dominant hand sterile and the nondominant hand nonsterile.			
8. Pours sterile saline into the sterile container using the nondominant hand.			
9. Picks up the suction catheter with the dominant hand and attaches it to the connection tubing, maintaining sterility of the hand and the catheter.			
10. Puts the tip of the suction catheter into the sterile container of normal saline solution and suctions a small amount of normal saline solution through the suction catheter. Applies suction by placing a finger over the suction control port of the suction catheter.			
11. Using the nondominant hand, removes the oxygen delivery device, if present.			
12. Has the patient take several slow deep breaths. If the patient's oxygen saturation is < 94%, or if he is in any distress, you may need to give supplemental oxygen before, during, and after suctioning. See Procedure Checklist Chapter 35: Administering Oxygen by Cannula, Face Mask, or Face Tent.			
13. Approximates the depth to insert the suction catheter (measures the distance between the tip of the			

PROCEDURE STEPS	Yes	No	COMMENTS
nose to the tip of the ear lobe and down to the bottom of the neck [for adults about 20 cm]); is careful not to contaminate the catheter while measuring.			
14. Lubricates the suction catheter tip with water-soluble lubricant.			
15. Using the dominant hand, gently but quickly inserts the suction catheter into the naris and down into the pharynx.			
16. Advances the suction catheter with inspiration to the predetermined distance, being careful not to force the catheter.			
17. Places a finger (thumb) over the suction control port of the catheter. Applies suction while withdrawing the catheter, using a continuous rotating motion.			
18. Applies suction for no longer than 10 seconds.			
19. After the catheter is withdrawn, clears it by placing the tip of the catheter into the container of sterile saline and applying suction.			
20. Lubricates the catheter and repeats suctioning as needed, allowing intervals of at least 30 seconds between suctioning. Reapplies oxygen between suctioning efforts, if required.			
21. Replaces the oxygen source.			
22. Coils the suction catheter in the dominant hand (alternatively, wraps it around the dominant hand). Holds the catheter while pulling the sterile glove off over it. Discards the glove containing the catheter in a water- resistant receptacle (e.g., bag) designated by the agency.			
23. Using the nondominant hand, clears the connecting tubing of secretions by placing the tip into the container of sterile saline.			
24. Disposes of equipment and makes sure new suction supplies are readily available for future suctioning.			
25. Provides mouth care.			

Recommendation: Pass _____ Needs more practice _____

Student: _____ Date: _____

Instructor: _____ Date: _____

Check (✓) Yes or No

PROCEDURE STEPS	Yes	No	COMMENTS
1. Positions the patient: a. <u>For oropharyngeal suctioning</u>: Semi-Fowler's position with his head turned toward the nurse. b. <u>Nasopharyngeal suctioning</u>: Semi-Fowler's position with his head hyperextended (unless contraindicated).			
2. Places the linen-saver pad or towel on the patient's chest.			
3. Puts on a face shield or goggles.			
4. Turns on the wall suction or portable suction machine and adjusts the pressure regulator according to policy (usually 100 to 120 mm Hg for adults, 95 to 110 mm Hg for children, and 50 to 95 mm Hg for infants).			
5. Tests the suction equipment by occluding the connection tubing.			
6. Opens the suction catheter kit or the gathered equipment if a kit is not available If using the nasal approach, opens the water-soluble lubricant.			
7. Dons sterile gloves; keeps the dominant hand sterile; considers nondominant hand nonsterile.			
8. Pours sterile saline into the sterile container, using the nondominant hand.			
9. Picks up the suction catheter with the dominant hand and attaches it to the connection tubing (to suction).			
10. Puts the tip of the suction catheter into the sterile container of normal saline solution and suctions a small amount of normal saline solution through the suction catheter. Applies suction by placing a finger over the suction control port.			
11. Approximates the depth to which to insert the suction catheter: a. <u>Oropharyngeal suctioning</u>: Measures the distance between the edge of the patient's mouth and the tip of the patient's ear lobe. b. <u>Nasopharyngeal suctioning</u>: Measures the distance between the tip of the patient's nose and the tip of the patient's ear lobe.			
12. Using the nondominant hand, removes the oxygen delivery device, if present. Has the patient take several slow deep breaths. If the patient's oxygen saturation is < 94%, or if he is in any distress, administers supplemental			

PROCEDURE STEPS	Yes	No	COMMENTS
oxygen before, during, and after suctioning. See Procedure Checklist Chapter 35: Administering Oxygen by Cannula, Face Mask, or Face Tent..			

13. Lubricates and inserts the suction catheter:
  a. Oropharyngeal suctioning
     1) Lubricates the catheter tip with normal saline.			

2) Using the dominant hand, gently but quickly inserts the suction catheter along the side of the patient's mouth into the oropharynx.			
3) Advances the suction catheter quickly to the premeasured distance (usually 7 to 10 cm in the adult), being careful not to force the catheter.			
b. Nasopharyngeal suctioning 1) Lubricates the catheter tip with the water-soluble lubricant.			
2) Using the dominant hand, gently but quickly inserts the suction catheter into the naris.			
3) Advances the suction catheter quickly to the premeasured distance (13 to 15 cm in the adult), being careful not to force the catheter.			
4) If resistance is met, tries using the other naris.			
14. Places a finger (thumb) over the suction control port of the suction catheter and starts suctioning the patient. Applies suction while withdrawing the catheter in a continuous rotating motion.			
15. Limits suctioning to 5 to 10 seconds.			
16. After the catheter is withdrawn, clears it by placing the tip of the catheter into the container of sterile saline and applying suction.			
17. Lubricates the catheter and repeats suctioning as needed, allowing at least 20-second intervals between suctioning. For nasopharyngeal suctioning, alternates nares each time suction is repeated.			
18. Coils the suction catheter in the dominant hand. Pulls the sterile glove off over the coiled catheter. (Alternatively, wraps the catheter around the dominant gloved hand and holds the catheter while removing the glove over it.)			

Recommendation: Pass _____ Needs more practice _____

Student: _____ Date: _____

Instructor: _____ Date: _____

Check (✓) Yes or No

PROCEDURE STEPS	Yes	No	COMMENTS
1. Positions the patient in semi-Fowler's position with his head turned facing the nurse.			
2. Places the linen-saver pad or towel on the patient's chest.			
3. Puts on a face shield or goggles.			
4. Turns on the wall suction or portable suction machine and adjusts the pressure regulator according to agency policy (typically 100 to 120 mm Hg for adults, 95 to 110 mm Hg for children, and 50 to 95 mm Hg for infants).			
5. Tests the suction equipment by occluding the connection tubing.			
6. Opens the suction catheter kit or the gathered equipment if a kit isn't available.			
7. Dons sterile gloves (alternatively, puts a sterile glove on the dominant hand and a clean procedure glove on the nondominant hand); considers the dominant hand sterile and the nondominant hand nonsterile.			
8. Pours sterile saline into the sterile container using the nondominant hand.			
9. Picks up the suction catheter with the dominant hand and attaches it to the connection tubing, maintaining sterility of the hand and the catheter.			
10.Puts the tip of the suction catheter into the sterile container of normal saline solution and suctions a small amount of normal saline solution through the suction catheter. Applies suction by placing a finger over the suction control port of the suction catheter.			
11. Using the nondominant hand, removes the oxygen delivery device, if present.			
12. Has the patient take several slow deep breaths. If the patient's oxygen saturation is < 94%, or if he is in any distress, you may need to give supplemental oxygen before, during, and after suctioning. See Procedure Checklist Chapter 35: Administering Oxygen by Cannula, Face Mask, or Face Tent.			
13. Approximates the depth to insert the suction catheter (measures distance between the edge of the mouth to the tip of the ear lobe and down to the bottom of the neck [for adults about 15 cm]); is careful not to contaminate the catheter while measuring.			

PROCEDURE STEPS	Yes	No	COMMENTS
14. Lubricates the suction catheter tip with normal saline.			
15. Using the dominant hand, gently but quickly inserts the suction catheter along the side of the patient's mouth into the oropharynx.			
16. Advances the suction catheter with inspiration to the predetermined distance, being careful not to force the catheter.			
17. Places a finger (thumb) over the suction control port of the catheter. Applies suction while withdrawing the catheter, using a continuous rotating motion.			
18. Applies suction for no longer than 10 seconds			
19. After the catheter is withdrawn, clears it by placing the tip of the catheter into the container of sterile saline and applying suction.			
20. Lubricates the catheter and repeats suctioning as needed, allowing intervals of at least 30 seconds between suctioning. Reapplies oxygen between suctioning efforts, if required.			
21. Replaces the oxygen source.			
22. Coils the suction catheter in the dominant hand (alternatively, wraps it around the dominant hand). Holds the catheter while pulling the sterile glove off over it. Discards the glove containing the catheter in a water resistant receptacle (e.g., bag) designated by the agency.			
23. Using the nondominant hand, clears the connecting tubing of secretions by placing the tip into the container of sterile saline.			
24. Disposes of equipment and makes sure new suction supplies are readily available for future suctioning.			
25. Provides mouth care.			

Recommendation: Pass _____ Needs more practice _____

Student: _____   Date: _____

Instructor: _____   Date: _____

Check (✓) Yes or No

PROCEDURE STEPS	Yes	No	COMMENTS
1. Helps the patient assume the appropriate position based on the lung field that requires drainage: a. <u>Apical areas of the upper lobes</u>: Has patient sit at the edge of the bed. Places a pillow at the base of the spine for support, if needed. If patient unable to sit at edge of the bed, places him in high Fowler's position. b. <u>Posterior section of the upper lobes</u>: Positions the patient in a supine position with pillow under his hips and knees flexed. Has the patient rotate slightly away from the side that requires drainage. c. <u>Middle or lower lobes</u>: Places the bed in Trendelenburg's position. Positions the patient in Sims' position. To drain the left lung, positions the patient on his right side. For the right lung, positions the patient on his left side. d. <u>Posterior lower lobes</u>: Keeping the bed flat, positions the patient prone with a pillow under his stomach.			
2. Has the patient remain in the desired position for 10 to 15 minutes.			
3. Performs percussion over the affected lung area while the patient is in the desired drainage position: a. Promotes relaxation by instructing the patient to breathe deeply and slowly.			
b. Covers the area to be percussed with a towel or the patient's gown.			
c. Avoids clapping over bony prominences, female breasts, or tender areas.			
d. Cups the hands, with fingers flexed and thumbs pressed against the index fingers.			
e. Places cupped hands over the lung area requiring drainage; percusses the area for 1 to 3 minutes by alternately striking cupped hands rhythmically against the patient.			

PROCEDURE STEPS	Yes	No	COMMENTS
4. Performs vibrations while the patient remains in the desired drainage position:			
a.. Places the flat surface of one hand over the lung area that requires vibration; places the other hand on top of that hand at a right angle.			
b. Instructs the patient to inhale slowly and deeply.			
c. Instructs the patient to make an "fff" or "sss" sound as he exhales.			
d. As the patient exhales, presses the fingers and palms firmly against the patient's chest wall and gently vibrates with the hands over the lung area.			
e. Continues performing vibrations for 3 exhalations.			
5. After performing postural drainage, percussion, and vibration, allows the patient to sit up. Has him cough at the end of a deep inspiration. Suctions the patient if he is unable to expectorate secretions.			
6. If a sputum specimen is needed, collects it in a specimen container.			
7. Repeats steps 1 through 5 for each lung field that requires treatment.			
8. The entire treatment does not exceed 60 minutes.			
9. Provides mouth care.			

Recommendation: Pass _____ Needs more practice _____

Student: _____   Date: _____

Instructor: _____   Date: _____

PROCEDURE CHECKLIST:
Chapter 35: Performing Tracheostomy Care

Check (✓) Yes or No

PROCEDURE STEPS	Yes	No	COMMENTS
1. Places the patient in semi-Fowler's position.			
2. Places a towel or linen-saver pad over the patient's chest.			
3. Dons sterile gloves (alternatively, puts a sterile glove on the dominant hand and a clean glove on the other hand).			
4. Suctions the tracheostomy (see Procedure Checklist Chapter 35: Performing Tracheostomy or Endotracheal Suctioning).			
5. Removes and discards the soiled tracheostomy dressing in a biohazard receptacle; then removes and discards gloves.			
6. Place the tracheostomy care equipment on the over-the-bed table and prepares the equipment using sterile technique:			
a. Pours hydrogen peroxide into one of the sterile solution containers and pours normal saline solution into the other one.			
b. Opens three 4×4 gauze packages; wets the gauze in one package with hydrogen peroxide; wets the gauze in another package with normal saline; keeps the third package dry.			
c. Opens 2 cotton-tipped applicator packages. Wets the applicators in one package with normal saline solution and wets the applicators in the other package with hydrogen peroxide.			
d. Opens the package containing a new disposable inner cannula, if available.			
e. Opens the package of Velcro tracheostomy ties or cuts a length of twill tape long enough to go around the patient's neck two times. Makes sure to cut end of the tape on an angle.			
7. Dons sterile gloves (or sterile on dominant and clean on nondominant hand); keeps the glove on the dominant hand sterile. Handles the sterile supplies with the dominant hand only.			

PROCEDURE STEPS	Yes	No	COMMENTS
8. With the nondominant hand removes the oxygen source, if the patient has been receiving supplemental oxygen.			
9. Unlocks and removes the inner cannula with the nondominant hand and cares for it accordingly: a. <u>Disposable Inner Cannula</u>: Disposes of the inner cannula in the biohazard receptacle according to agency policy. b. <u>Reusable Inner Cannula</u>: Places the inner cannula into the basin filled with hydrogen peroxide.			
10. Attaches the oxygen source to the outer cannula, if possible.			
11. Cares for the inner cannula: a. <u>Variation: Disposable Inner Cannula</u>: Picks up the new disposable inner cannula, holding it by the outer locking portion.			
b. <u>Reusable Inner Cannula</u>: 1) Picks up the reusable inner cannula from the container of hydrogen peroxide and scrubs it with the sterile nylon brush, using the dominant hand. 2) Immerses the inner cannula in the container of sterile normal saline and agitates it until it is thoroughly rinsed. 3) Taps the inner cannula against the side of the container to remove excess fluid.			
12. Removes the oxygen source, using nondominant hand, (if the patient requires supplemental oxygen) and reinserts the inner cannula into the patient's tracheostomy in the direction of the curvature.			
13. Following manufacturer instructions, locks the inner cannula in place securely.			
14. Reattaches the oxygen source, if indicated.			
15. Cleans the stoma under the faceplate with the cotton-tipped applicators saturated with hydrogen peroxide, using a circular motion from the stoma site outward.			
16. Uses each applicator only once and then discards it.			

PROCEDURE STEPS	Yes	No	COMMENTS
17. Cleans the top surface of the faceplate and the skin around it with the gauze pads saturated with hydrogen peroxide. Uses each gauze pad only once, and then discards it.			
18. Repeats steps 15, 16, and 17, using the cotton-tipped applicators and gauze pads saturated with normal saline.			
19. Dries the skin and outer cannula surfaces by patting them lightly with the remaining dry gauze pads.			
20. Removes soiled tracheostomy stabilizers: a. Variation: Velcro Tracheostomy Holder: With an assistant stabilizing the tracheostomy tube, disengages the Velcro on both sides of the soiled holder and removes it gently from the eyes of the faceplate. Discards the Velcro holder in the nearest biohazard receptacle. b. Variation: Twill Tape Tracheostomy Ties: With the assistant stabilizing the tracheostomy tube, cuts the soiled tracheostomy ties using bandage scissors. Avoids cutting the tube of the tracheostomy balloon. Removes the ties gently from the eyes of the faceplate and discards them in the nearest biohazard receptacle.			
21. Has the patient flex his neck and applies new tracheostomy stabilizers.			
a. Variation: Velcro Tracheostomy Holder: 1) Unfastens the Velcro; threads one end of the tracheostomy holder through the eyelet of the faceplate, and fastens the Velcro.			
2) Brings the holder around the back of the patient's neck and threads the remaining end of the tracheostomy holder through the empty eyelet of the faceplate. Fastens the Velcro, making sure the holder fits securely.			
3) Places one finger under the holder to make sure the holder is securing the tracheostomy effectively, but is not too tight.			
b. Variation: Using Twill Tape: 1) Threads one end of the twill tape into one of the eyelets on the tracheostomy faceplate; continues to thread the twill tape through the eyelet, bringing both ends of the tape together.			

PROCEDURE STEPS	Yes	No	COMMENTS
2) Brings both ends of the twill tape around the back of the patient's neck.			
3) Threads the end of the twill tape that is closest to the patient's neck through the back of the eyelet on the faceplate.			
4) Has the assistant place one finger under the tape while tying the two ends together in a square knot.			
22. Inserts a precut, sterile tracheostomy dressing under the faceplate and new tracheostomy stabilizers.			
23. Disposes of used equipment/supplies in the appropriate biohazard receptacle, according to agency policy.			

Recommendation: Pass _____ Needs more practice _____

Student: _____ Date: _____

Instructor: _____ Date: _____

Check (✓) Yes or No

PROCEDURE STEPS	Yes	No	COMMENTS
1. Positions the patient in semi-Fowler's position, unless contraindicated.			
2. Places a linen-saver pad or towel on the patient's chest.			
3. Puts on a face shield or goggles.			
4. Turns on the wall suction or portable suction machine and adjusts the pressure regulator according to agency policy (typically 100 to 120 mm Hg for adults, 95 to 110 mm Hg for children, and 50 to 95 mm Hg for infants).			
5. Tests the suction equipment by occluding the connection tubing.			
6. Opens the suction catheter kit or the gathered equipment if a kit is not available.			
7. Dons sterile gloves. Considers the dominant hand sterile and the nondominant hand nonsterile.			
8. Pours sterile saline into the sterile container, using the nondominant hand.			
9. Picks up the suction catheter with the dominant hand and attaches it to the connection tubing.			
10. Puts the tip of the suction catheter into the sterile container of normal saline solution and suctions a small amount of normal saline solution through the catheter. Applies suction by placing a finger over the suction control port of the suction catheter.			
11. Hyperoxygenates the patient according to agency policy: a. Patient Requiring Mechanical Ventilation: Presses the 100% O_2 button on the ventilator or attaches the resuscitation bag to the endotracheal tube or tracheostomy tube and manually hyperoxygenates the patient by compressing the resuscitation bag 3 to 5 times as the patient inhales. Removes the resuscitation bag and places it next to the patient when finished.			

PROCEDURE STEPS	Yes	No	COMMENTS
b. <u>Patient Not Requiring Mechanical Ventilation:</u> Attaches the resuscitation bag to the tracheostomy or endotracheal tube and hyperoxygenates the patient by compressing the resuscitation bag 3 to 5 times. Removes the resuscitation bag and places it next to the patient when finished.			
12. Lubricates the suction catheter tip with normal saline.			
13. Using the dominant hand, gently but quickly inserts the suction catheter into the endotracheal tube or tracheostomy tube.			
14. Advances the suction catheter, with suction off, gently aiming downward and being careful not to force the catheter.			
15. Applies suction while withdrawing the catheter.			
16. Does not apply suction for longer than 10 seconds.			
17. Repeats suctioning as needed, allowing at least 30-second intervals between suctioning.			
18. Hyperoxygenates patient between each pass.			
19. Replaces the oxygen source, if the patient was removed from the source during suctioning.			
20. Coils the suction catheter in the dominant hand (alternatively, wraps it around the dominant hand). Pulls the sterile glove off over the coiled catheter.			
21. Discards the glove and catheter in a water resistant receptacle designated by the agency.			
22. Using the nondominant hand, clears the connecting tubing of secretions by placing the tip into the container of sterile saline.			
23. Provides mouth care.			

<u>Recommendation</u>: Pass _____ Needs more practice _____

Student: _____   Date: _____

Instructor: _____   Date: _____

PROCEDURE CHECKLIST
**Chapter 35: Performing Tracheostomy or Endotracheal Suctioning Using
Inline Suctioning Equipment**

Check (✓) Yes or No

PROCEDURE STEPS	Yes	No	COMMENTS
1. Prepares the equipment. An in-line suction unit is only available for patients on a mechanical ventilator. Most agencies require the respiratory therapy department to setup the in-line suction equipment. If this is not your agency's policy, performs the following to prepare equipment for future use. These steps need to be performed only one time per day.			
a. Opens the in-line suction catheter using sterile technique.			
b. Removes the adapter on the ventilator tubing.			
c. Attaches the in-line suction catheter equipment to the ventilator tubing.			
d. Reconnects the adapter on the ventilator tubing.			
e. Attaches the other end of the in-line suction catheter to the connection tubing.			
2. Positions the patient in semi-Fowler's position, unless contraindicated.			
3. Places linen-saver pad or towel on patient's chest.			
4. Puts on face shield or goggles.			
5. Turns on the wall suction or portable suction machine and adjusts the pressure regulator according to agency policy (typically 100 to 120 mm Hg for adults, 95 to 110 mm Hg for children, and 50 to 95 mm Hg for infants).			
6. Hyperoxygenates the patient according to agency policy.			
7. Dons clean procedure gloves.			
8. If a lock is present on the suction control port, unlocks it.			
9. With the dominant hand, picks up the suction catheter contained within the plastic sleeve.			
10. Gently inserts the suction catheter into the airway by maneuvering the catheter within the sterile sleeve.			
11. Advances the suction catheter into the airway, being careful not to force the catheter. Advances the catheter until meeting resistance.			

PROCEDURE STEPS	Yes	No	COMMENTS
12. Applies suction by depressing the button over the suction control port, while withdrawing the catheter. Makes sure to apply suction for no longer than 10 seconds.			
13. Withdraws the in-line suction catheter completely into the sleeve. The indicator line on the catheter should appear through the sleeve.			
14. Attaches the prefilled, 10-mL container of normal saline solution to the saline port located on the in-line equipment.			
15. Squeezes the 10-mL container of normal saline while applying suction.			
16. Locks the suction regulator port.			

Recommendation: Pass _____ Needs more practice _____

Student: _____   Date: _____

Instructor: _____   Date: _____

PROCEDURE CHECKLIST
Chapter 36: Administering a Blood Transfusion

Check (✓) Yes or No

PROCEDURE STEPS	Yes	No	COMMENTS
1. Verifies that informed consent has been obtained.			
2. Verifies the physician's order, noting the indication, rate of infusion, and any premedication orders.			
3. Administers any pretransfusion medications as prescribed.			
4. Obtains IV fluid containing normal saline solution and a blood administration set.			
5. Obtains the blood product from the blood bank according to agency policy.			
6. Wears procedure gloves whenever handling blood products.			
7. Rechecks the physician's order.			
8. With another qualified staff member (as deemed by the institution) verifies the patient and blood product identification, as follows:			
a. Has the patient state his full name and date of birth (if he is able) and compares it to the name and date of birth located on the blood bank form.			
b. Compares the patient name and hospital identification number on the patient's identification bracelet with the patient name and hospital identification number on the blood bank form attached to the blood product.			
c. Compares the unit identification number located on the blood bank form with the identification number printed on the blood product container.			
d. Compares the patient's blood type listed on the blood bank form with the blood type listed on the blood product container.			
e. If all verifications are in agreement, both staff members sign the blood bank form attached to the blood product container. Contacts the blood bank immediately if any discrepancies occur during the identification process; and does not administer the blood product.			
f. Documents on the blood bank form the date and time that the transfusion was begun.			
g. Makes sure that the blood bank form remains attached to the blood product container until administration is complete.			
9. Removes the blood administration set from the package and labels the tubing with the date and time.			

PROCEDURE STEPS	Yes	No	COMMENTS
10. Closes the clamps on the administration set.			
11. Removes the protective covers from the normal saline solution container port and one of the spikes located on the "Y" of the blood product administration set. Places the spike into the port of the solution container and opens the roller clamp closest to that spike.			
12. Hangs the normal saline solution container on the IV pole.			
13. Compresses the drip chamber of the administration set and allows it to fill up half way.			
14. Primes the administration set with normal saline.			
15. Attaches the blood filter to the second "Y" port on the administration set and primes it with normal saline solution by inverting it.			
16. Inspects the tubing for air. If air bubbles remain in the tubing, flicks the tubing with a fingernail to mobilize the bubbles.			
17. Gently inverts the blood product container several times.			
18. Removes the protective covers from the administration set and the blood product port. Carefully spikes the blood product container through the port.			
19. Hangs the blood product container on the IV pole.			
20. Slowly opens the roller clamp closest to the blood product.			
21. Obtains and records the patient's vital signs, including temperature, before beginning the transfusion.			
22. Using aseptic technique, attaches the distal end of the administration set to the IV catheter.			
23. Using the roller clamp, adjusts the drip rate, as prescribed. (Keep in mind that blood administration sets have a drip factor of 10 drops/mL.).			
24. Remains with the patient during the first 5 minutes and then obtains vital signs.			
25. Makes sure that the patient's call bell or light is readily available and tells him alert the nurse immediately of any signs or symptoms of a transfusion reaction, such as back pain, chills, itching, or shortness of breath.			
26. Obtains vital signs in 15 minutes, then again in 30 minutes, and then hourly while the transfusion infuses.			
27. After the unit has infused, closes the roller clamp closest to the blood product container and opens the roller clamp closest to the normal saline solution to flush the			

PROCEDURE STEPS	Yes	No	COMMENTS
administration set with normal saline solution.			
28. Closes the roller clamp and then disconnects the blood administration set from the IV catheter.			
29. If another unit of blood is required, the second unit can be hung with the same administration set.			
30. Discards the empty blood container and administration set in the proper receptacle according to agency policy.			
Variation A: Transfusion Reaction			
31. Stops the transfusion immediately if signs or symptoms of a transfusion reaction occur.			
32. Does not flush the tubing with the normal saline solution attached to the blood administration set.			
33. Disconnects the administration set from the IV catheter.			
34. Obtains vital signs and auscultates heart and breath sounds.			
35. Maintains a patent IV catheter by hanging a new infusion of normal saline solution, using new tubing.			
36. Notifies physician as soon as the blood has been stopped and patient has been assessed.			
37. Places the administration set and blood product container with the blood bank form attached inside a biohazard bag and sends it to the blood bank immediately.			
38. Obtains blood (in the extremity opposite the transfusion site) and urine specimens according to agency policy.			
39. Continues to monitor vital signs frequently.			
40. Administers medications as prescribed.			

Recommendation: Pass _____ Needs more practice _____

Student: _____   Date: _____

Instructor: _____   Date: _____

PROCEDURE CHECKLIST
Chapter 36: Changing IV Solutions, Tubing, and Dressings

Check (✓) Yes or No

PROCEDURE STEPS	Yes	No	COMMENTS
Changing the IV Solution			
1. Using the six rights of medication administration, prepares and labels the next container of IV solution 1 hour before the present infusion is scheduled for completion.			
2. Closes the roller clamp on the administration set.			
3. Wearing procedure gloves, removes the old IV solution container from the IV pole. Removes the spike from the bag, keeping the spike sterile.			
4. Removes the protective cover from the new IV solution container port. Places the spike into the port of the new solution container. If the solution is contained in a glass IV bottle, first cleans the rubber stopper on the top of the bottle with an alcohol pad; then, inserts the spike of the administration set through the rubber stopper.			
5. Hangs the IV solution container on the IV pole.			
6. Inspects the tubing to be sure it is free of air bubbles and the drip chamber remains half filled.			
7. Opens the roller clamp, and adjusts the drip rate, as prescribed.			
8. Affixes the time tape to the new IV solution container. Marks the tape with the time the infusion was started and continues to mark 1-hour intervals on the time tape until reaching the bottom of the container.			
Changing the IV Administration Tubing and Solution			
9. Using the six rights of medication administration, prepares and labels the next container of IV solution 1 hour before the present infusion is scheduled for completion.			
10. Wearing procedure gloves, carefully removes the tape securing the catheter tubing connection.			
11. Closes the roller clamp on the old administration set.			
12. Hangs the new administration set on the IV pole.			
13. Removes the protective cover from the distal end of the new administration set.			
14. Stabilizes the IV catheter with the nondominant hand while applying pressure over the vein just above the insertion site.			

PROCEDURE STEPS	Yes	No	COMMENTS
15. Quickly, but gently, disengages the old tubing from the IV catheter and inserts the new tubing into the IV catheter. Uses a hemostat ("mosquito" clamp) to hold the catheter hub if old tubing does not loosen easily.			
16. Opens the roller clamp on the new administration set and allows the IV solution to infuse.			
17. Using the roller clamp, adjusts the flow until the prescribed rate is achieved.			
18. Resecures the IV catheter and tubing connection.			
Changing the IV Dressing			
19. Wearing procedure gloves, stabilizes the catheter with nondominant hand and carefully removes dressing.			
20. Inspects the insertion site for erythema, drainage, and tenderness. Removes IV if present.			
21. Using a circular motion, cleanses the insertion site with an antiseptic swab containing 2% tincture of iodine, alcohol, or chlorhexidine. (Avoids using chlorhexidine in infants under age 2 months.) Starts at the insertion site and works outward several inches.			
22. Allows the antiseptic to dry on the skin.			
23. Covers the insertion site with a sterile semipermeable transparent dressing. a. Opens the package containing the dressing. Remove the protective backing from the dressing making sure not to touch the sterile surface.			
b. Covers the insertion site and the hub or winged portion of the catheter with the dressing. Does not cover the tubing of the administration set.			
c. Gently pinches the transparent dressing around the catheter hub to secure the hub.			
d. Smoothes the remainder of the dressing so that it adheres to the skin.			
24. Loops the administration tubing and places a piece of tape over the catheter tubing connection and looped section of tubing.			
25. Labels the dressing with the date and time of insertion, catheter size, and initials.			

Recommendation: Pass _____ Needs more practice _____

Student: _____   Date: _____

Instructor: _____   Date: _____

PROCEDURE CHECKLIST
Chapter 36: Converting a Primary Line to a Heparin or Saline Lock

Check (✓) Yes or No

PROCEDURE STEPS	Yes	No	COMMENTS
1. Helps the client assume a comfortable position that provides access to his IV site.			
2. Places a linen-saver pad under the extremity with the IV catheter.			
3. Applies procedure gloves.			
4. Removes the IV lock from the package and flushes the adapter with the first syringe (of saline or dilute heparin, according to unit policy); places the lock back loosely inside the sterile package.			
5. Carefully removes the IV dressing and the tape that is securing the tubing.			
6. Closes the roller clamp on the administration set.			
7. With the nondominant hand applies pressure over the vein just above the insertion site.			
8. Gently disengages the old tubing from the IV catheter. If it does not disengage easily, grips the catheter hub with a hemostat (small "mosquito" clamp).			
9. Quickly inserts the lock adapter into the IV catheter.			
10. Cleanses the injection port of the adapter with an alcohol pad.			
11. Inserts a syringe containing saline or dilute heparin into the injection port of the adapter. Flushes the catheter gently with the solution.			
12. Covers the insertion site with a sterile transparent semipermeable dressing.			
a. Opens the package containing the dressing. Using aseptic technique, removes the protective backing from the dressing making sure not to touch the sterile surface.			
b. Covers the insertion site and the hub or winged portion of the catheter with the dressing. Does not cover the tubing of the administration set.			
c. Gently pinches the transparent dressing around the catheter hub to secure the hub.			
d. Smoothes the remainder of the dressing so that it adheres to the skin.			
13. Discards the administration set and linen-saver pad in the appropriate receptacle, as designated by the agency.			
14. Empties the IV solution container in the nearest sink and then discards it appropriately.			

PROCEDURE STEPS	Yes	No	COMMENTS

Recommendation: Pass _____ Needs more practice _____

Student: _____   Date: _____

Instructor: _____   Date: _____

PROCEDURE CHECKLIST
Chapter 36: Discontinuing an IV Line

Check (✓) Yes or No

PROCEDURE STEPS	Yes	No	COMMENTS
1. Assists the client to a comfortable position.			
2. Places a linen-saver pad under the extremity that contains the IV catheter.			
3. Applies procedure gloves.			
4. Closes the roller clamp on the administration set.			
5. Carefully removes the IV dressing and tape that is securing the tubing.			
6. Applies a sterile 2×2 gauze pad above the IV insertion site and gently removes the catheter, directing it straight along the vein. Does not press down on the gauze pad while removing the catheter.			
7. Immediately applies firm pressure with the gauze pad over the insertion site. Holds pressure for 2 to 3 minutes; longer if bleeding persists.			
8. Removes the soiled 2×2 gauze pad and replaces it with a sterile 2×2 gauze pad. Secures it with a piece of 1-inch tape.			
9. Disposes of the IV catheter in the appropriate sharps container.			
10. Discards the IV tubing, linen-saver pad, IV solution container, and gloves in the appropriate trash container, according to agency policy.			

Recommendation: Pass _____ Needs more practice _____

Student: _____   Date: _____

Instructor: _____   Date: _____

PROCEDURE CHECKLIST
Chapter 36: Initiating a Peripheral Intravenous Infusion

Check (✓) Yes or No

PROCEDURE STEPS	Yes	No	COMMENTS
1. Prepares the intravenous solution and administration set.			
a. Utilizing the six rights of medication administration, checks the IV solution to make sure it is the proper solution with the prescribed additives.			
b. Checks the expiration date on the IV solution bag.			
c. Checks solution for discoloration or particulate matter.			
d. Labels the IV solution container with the patient's name, date, and own initials.			
e. Places a time tape on the solution container with the prescribed infusion rate, time the infusion began, and the time of completion.			
f. Takes the administration set from the package, labels the tubing with the date and time, and then closes the roller clamp.			
g. Removes the protective cover from the IV solution container port.			
h. Removes the protective cover from the spike on the IV administration set, making sure the spike remains sterile. Places the spike into the port of the solution container. If the solution is in a glass bottle, first cleans the rubber stopper on the top of the bottle with an alcohol pad, then inserts the spike through the rubber stopper.			
i. Makes certain the tubing is clamped; hangs the IV solution container on an IV pole.			
j. Lightly compresses the drip chamber and allows it to fill up halfway. If using extension tubing, attaches it to the end of the administration set.			
k. Primes the tubing by opening the roller clamp and allowing the fluid to slowly fill the tubing.			
l. Inspects the tubing for air. If air bubbles remain in the tubing, flicks the tubing with a fingernail to mobilize the bubbles. Recaps end of tubing firmly.			

PROCEDURE STEPS	Yes	No	COMMENTS
2. Locates a vein for inserting the IV catheter. Selects the most distal vein on the hand or arm. Avoids using an arm or hand that contains a dialysis graft or fistula or the affected arm of a mastectomy patient.			
3. Places a linen-saver pad under the patient's arm.			
4. Places the patient's arm in a dependent position and applies a tourniquet 4 to 6 inches above the selected site.			
5. Palpates the radial pulse; if no pulse is present, loosens the tourniquet and reapplies it with less tension.			
6. Palpates the vein and presses it downward, making sure that it rebounds quickly. If the vein is not adequately dilated, has the patient open and close his fist, applies heat (e.g., a warm towel), lightly taps the vein site, or strokes the extremity from distal to proximal below the selected venipuncture site.			
7. After selecting the vein, gently releases the tourniquet.			
8. If excessive hair is present at the venipuncture site, clips it with a scissor.			
9. Applies procedure gloves.			
10. Chooses an appropriate IV catheter based on the size of the vein and the solution to be infused.			
11. Using aseptic technique, opens the catheter package.			
12. Gently reapplies the tourniquet and cleanses the site, using an antiseptic swab that contains 2% tincture of iodine, alcohol, or chlorhexidine. (Avoid using chlorhexidine in infants under age 2 months.)			
13. Cleanses the area using a circular motion starting at the site and working outward several inches.			
14. Allows the antiseptic to dry on the skin.			
15. Using the nondominant hand, stabilizes the vein by stretching the skin over the vein, making sure not to contaminate the insertion site.			
16. Informs the patient that he is about to insert the catheter and that it may be uncomfortable.			

PROCEDURE STEPS	Yes	No	COMMENTS

17. Picks up the catheter:
 	
  a. <u>Wing-tipped (butterfly) catheter</u>: Grasps the catheter by the wings, using the thumb and forefinger of the dominant hand—bevel up; removes protective cap from the needle.
  b. <u>Over-the-needle catheter</u>: Grasps the catheter by the hub, using the thumb and forefinger of the dominant hand—bevel up.			

18. Holding the catheter at a 20- to 30-degree angle, pierces the skin.			
19. Lowers the catheter so that it is parallel to the skin and advances the catheter into the vein. Watches for a flashback of blood into the chamber of the catheter or the tubing of the winged catheter.			

20. Advances catheter:
 	
  a. <u>Wing-tipped catheter</u>: Fully advances the catheter.
  b. <u>Over-the-needle catheter</u>: Advances the catheter to half its length. Withdraws the needle while advancing the catheter fully into the vein.			

21. While holding the catheter in place with one hand, releases the tourniquet with the other hand.			
22. Quickly connects the administration set adapter to IV catheter, using aseptic technique.			
23. Still stabilizing the catheter, slowly opens the roller clamp and allows the IV fluid to flush the catheter. Adjusts the flow rate according to the physician's order.			
24. Covers the insertion site with a sterile semipermeable transparent dressing. If the site isn't clean and dry, cleans the site with an antiseptic swab and allows it to dry before applying the dressing.			
a. Opens the package containing the dressing. Using aseptic technique, removes the protective backing from the dressing making sure not to touch the sterile surface.			
b. Covers the insertion site and the hub or winged portion of the catheter with the dressing. Does not cover the tubing of the administration set.			
c. Gently pinches the transparent dressing around the catheter hub to secure the hub.			
d. Smoothes the remainder of the dressing so that it adheres to the skin.			

PROCEDURE STEPS	Yes	No	COMMENTS
25. Loops the administration tubing and places a piece of tape over the catheter tubing connection, and looped section of tubing.			
26. Labels the dressing with the date and time of insertion, catheter size, and own initials.			
27. If the insertion site is located near a joint, places an arm board under the joint and secures it with tape.			

Recommendation: Pass _____ Needs more practice _____

Student: _____   Date: _____

Instructor: _____   Date: _____

PROCEDURE CHECKLIST
Chapter 36: Regulating the IV Flow Rate

Check (✓) Yes or No

PROCEDURE STEPS	Yes	No	COMMENTS
1. Uses the six rights of medication administration. Checks the solution to make sure that the proper IV fluid is hanging with the prescribed additives. Also verifies the infusion rate.			
2. Calculates the hourly rate if it is not specified in the order. (Divides the volume to be infused by the number of hours it is to be infused. For example if the physician prescribes 1,000 mL to run over 4 hours, the infusion rate is 250 mL/hour).			
3. Calculates the drip rate by multiplying the number of mL to be infused in 60 minutes by the drop factor in drops/mL; then divides by 60 minutes: Hourly rate in mL × drop factor = drip rate 60 minutes			
4. Verifies calculations.			
5. Applies a time tape to the IV solution container next to the volume markings. Marks the time tape with the time that the infusion was started. Continues to mark 1-hour intervals on the time tape until reaching the bottom of the container.			
6. Opens the roller clamp so that the IV fluid begins to flow.			
7. Using a watch, counts the number of drops entering the drip chamber in 1 minute.			
8. Adjusts the roller clamp by increasing or decreasing the flow until the prescribed drip rate is achieved.			
9. Monitors the infusion rate 15 minutes after the infusion is begun; then monitors hourly.			

Recommendation: Pass _____ Needs more practice _____

Student: _____ Date: _____

Instructor: _____ Date: _____

PROCEDURE CHECKLIST
Chapter 36: Setting Up and Using IV Pumps

Check (✓) Yes or No

PROCEDURE STEPS	Yes	No	COMMENTS
1. Calculates the hourly infusion rate by dividing the volume to be infused by the number of hours it is to be infused.			
2. Verifies the calculation.			
3. Attaches the IV pump to the IV pole and plugs it in to the nearest electrical outlet.			
4. Takes the administration set from the package; labels the tubing with the date and time.			
5. Closes the clamp on the administration set.			
6. Removes the protective covers and spikes the port of the solution container with the administration set.			
7. Hangs the IV solution container on the IV pole.			
8. Compresses the drip chamber of the administration set and allows it to fill up halfway.			
9. Places the electronic eye on the drip chamber between the fluid level and the origin of the drop (if there is no electronic eye, consults the manufacturers instructions for setup).			
10. If a filter is required, attaches it to the end of the administration set.			
11. Primes the administration set with fluid by opening the roller clamp and allowing the fluid to flow slowly through the tubing. Closes the clamp.			
12. Inspects the tubing for the presence of air. If air bubbles remain in the tubing, flicks the tubing with a fingernail to mobilize the bubbles.			
13. Turns on the IV pump and loads the administration tubing into the pump according to manufacturer's instructions.			
14. Programs the pump with the prescribed infusion rate (hourly rate) and the volume to be infused (usually the total amount in the IV bag).			
15. Applies procedure gloves and connects the administration set adapter to the IV catheter.			
16. Unclamps the administration set tubing (opens roller clamp all the way) and presses the "start" button on the pump.			
17. Ensures that all alarms are turned on and audible.			

PROCEDURE STEPS	Yes	No	COMMENTS
18. Checks the pump hourly to make sure the correct volume is infusion.			
19. At end of shift (or at the time specified by the agency), clears the pump of the volume infused and records the volume on the I&O form.			

Recommendation: Pass _____ Needs more practice _____

Student: _____ Date: _____

Instructor: _____ Date: _____

PROCEDURE CHECKLIST
Chapter 37: Applying Antiembolism Stockings

Check (✓) Yes or No

PROCEDURE STEPS	Yes	No	COMMENTS
1. Ensures that patient lies supine for at least 15 minutes prior to stocking application.			
2. Measures extremity; obtains correct size stockings.			
a. Thigh-High Stockings			
1) Measures the circumference of the thigh at the widest section.			
2) Measures the calf circumference at the widest section.			
3) Measures the distance from the gluteal fold to the base of the heel.			
b. Knee-High Stockings			
1) Measures the circumference of the calf at the widest section.			
2) Measures the distance from the base of the heel to the middle of the knee joint.			
3. Cleanses patient's legs and feet if necessary. Dries well.			
4. Lightly dusts legs and feet with talcum powder, if available, desired, appropriate for patient, and recommended by manufacturer.			
5. Holds top cuff in dominant hand, slides nondominant arm into stocking until hand reaches stocking heel; turns stocking inside out, stopping when the heel reaches the level of the dominant hand.			
6. Grasps the heel with hand still inside the turned ("bunched") stocking and, having the patient point his toes, eases the stocking onto patient's foot.			
7. Centers patients heel in the heel of the stocking.			
8. Pulls stocking up to 1 to 2 inches below the knee or to the gluteal fold (depending on stocking type).			
9. Stocking is straight and free of wrinkles.			
10. Tugs on stocking toe to create a small space between end of toes and stocking.			
11. Repeats procedure on the other leg.			

Recommendation: Pass _____ Needs more practice _____

Student: _____   Date: _____

Instructor: _____   Date: _____

PROCEDURE CHECKLIST
Chapter 37: Applying Sequential Compression Devices

Check (✓) Yes or No

PROCEDURE STEPS	Yes	No	COMMENTS
1. Cleanses patient's legs and feet, if necessary.			
2. Applies elastic stockings if they are ordered in conjunction with the SCD.			
3. Measures extremity following manufacturer's instructions; obtains proper size sleeve.			
4. Places patient supine.			
5. Places SCD pump in a safe location and plugs it in.			
6. Applies compression sleeve correctly:			
a. *For "Flowtron" brand sleeves (knee-length only):* 1) Opens the Velcro fasteners on the sleeve.			
2) Places the sleeve under the lower leg below the knee, with the "air bladder" side down on the bed.			
3) Brings the ends of the sleeve up and wraps around the lower leg, leaving 1–2 fingerbreadths of space between the leg and the sleeve.			
b. *For SCDS/PAS brand sleeves:* 1) Opens Velcro fasteners on the sleeve and places the sleeve under the leg, ensuring that the fastener will close on the anterior surface.			
2) For thigh-high sleeves: Places the opened sleeve under the leg, ensuring that the knee opening is at the level of the knee joint.			
3) Brings the ends of the sleeve up and wraps around the lower leg, leaving 1–2 fingerbreadths of space between the leg and the sleeve. Wraps upper leg similarly.			
7. Connects sleeve to compression pump.			
8. Turns pump on.			
9. Sets compression pressure, if applicable, to manufacturer's recommended setting.			

Recommendation: Pass _____ Needs more practice _____

Student: _____   Date: _____

Instructor: _____   Date: _____

Check (✓) Yes or No

PROCEDURE STEPS	Yes	No	COMMENTS
Teaching a Patient to Cough and Deep-Breathe			
1. Assists patient to assume Fowler's or semi-Fowler's position.			
2. For a patient with chest or abdominal incision, provides and demonstrates splinting with blanket or pillow.			

3. <u>Diaphragmatic breathing</u>. Tells patient to:
    a. Place hands anteriorly along lower rib cage, third fingers touching at midline.
    b. Take deep breath slowly through the nose, feeling the chest expand.
    c. Hold her breath for 2 to 5 seconds, then exhale slowly and completely through the mouth.			

4. <u>Coughing</u>. Tells patient to:
    a. Complete 2 or 3 cycles of diaphragmatic breathing.
    b. On the next breath, lean forward and cough several times through an open mouth.
    c. If the patient is too weak to cough, has patient inhale deeply and perform three or four huffs against an open glottis.			

Teaching a Patient to Move in Bed			
1. Positions patient supine, bed rails up.			

2. Instructs patient to (when turning left):
    a. Bend right leg, sliding foot flat along the bed and flexing knee.
    b. Reach right arm across the chest and grab the opposite bedrail.
    c. Take a deep breath, splinting any abdominal or chest incisions.
    d. Pull on the bedrail while pushing off with right foot.			

3. If patient cannot maintain position independently, places pillow or blanket along back for support.			
Teaching the Patient Leg Exercises			
1. Positions patient supine.			

PROCEDURE STEPS	Yes	No	COMMENTS
2. <u>Ankle Circles</u>. Instructs patient to: 　a. Start with one foot in the dorsiflexed position. 　b. Slowly rotate the ankle clockwise. 　c. After three rotations, repeat the procedure in a counterclockwise direction. 　d. Repeat this exercise at least three times in each direction, then switch and exercise the other ankle.			
3. <u>Ankle Pumps</u>. Instructs patient to: 　a. With leg extended, point the toe until her foot is plantar flexed. 　b. Pull the toes back toward her head until the foot is dorsiflexed; at the same time, press the back of the knee into the bed. 　c. Make sure she feels a "pull" in the calf. 　d. Repeat the alternate plantar and dorsiflexion several times. 　e. Repeat the cycle with the other foot.			
4. <u>Leg Exercises</u>. Instructs patient to: 　a. Slowly begin bending the knee, sliding the sole of the foot along the bed until the knee is in a flexed position. 　b. Reverse the motion, extending the knee until the leg is once again flat on the bed. 　c. Repeat several times. 　d. Repeat using the opposite leg.			

<u>Recommendation</u>: Pass _____ Needs more practice _____

Student: _____　　　Date: _____

Instructor: _____　　　Date: _____